My Simple Changes

COOKBOOK

BY
BRANDON GODSEY

TABLE OF CONTENTS

ABOUT ME

———————

Welcome. To your first change. Yeah, that's right. Because by opening this book you made the conscious choice to improve your health, and because of that, you will.

To start this off, we have to address the elephant in the room: This world around us is not set up for our success. Toxins load our every day and weigh us a little more with every substance's consumption. Capitalism has made access to everything seem endless. The need for profits and a decreased bottom line have clouded our clarity. So much that what were once known as rare autoimmune conditions have now reached most of us in one way or another. Our immune systems are broken. Our lifestyles are too fast for our own good. Our susceptibility to viruses and diseases is greater than ever.

I'm here to tell you that this doesn't have to be the case. Not anymore. Not when the solutions are real, the food is still delicious, the price is the same, and success can be had.

Let's go back to my beginnings. From nearly the time I was born, I've been fighting illnesses. Each sickness wearing me down a little more and the next condition getting a little worse, when all I ever wanted was to just be healthy. I've also always enjoyed helping others, being an artist, and finding relief from ailments in doing whatever it took to make people laugh. After decades of me hiding in laughter, medicine, and a reckless lifestyle came the diagnosis of the autoimmune condition, Crohn's disease. A few years after, having ignored all the warning signs, I had eighteen inches of my intestine removed. A few years later, after still carrying on with the same habits, my infusion medicine caused a horrible case of shingles. It was then, after nearly thirty years of pain, bloody stools, frustration, depression, surgeries, poor diet, no answers, one pill solutions, and a toxic lifestyle, that I decided to finally find my own smiles, or solutions. Letting go of the dependency and helping the person who needed it the most.

This self-taught approach evolved from my experience and slowly grew through five years of reading every label, researching every ingredient, and understanding all aspects of how the body functions. Eventually I heard the words that everyone suffering from illness deserves to hear: "no active disease."

That was a special day. I was elated, relieved, proud, and right. I was also angry. So, so angry. I was angry because I always knew I had the will to heal, but it took that long to give myself the permission. After that day, I again resorted to creative therapy and started to write down my story and methods. To resolve my unresolved, and to pay it forward so you can heal, too. After the bestselling success of *My Simple Changes* and the audiobook that followed comes this, the next tool for your new foundation: the cookbook.

This book contains snippets of what I've learned, quotes of the inspiration I've held, and carefully designed recipes I have formulated. It also includes ingredients, supplements, cookware, budget tactics, and strategies that I used from my final infusion treatment until now. Everything is separated into three phases: the calming phase, the expansion phase, and the reintroduction phase. Each phase is structured to provide relief for the next expansion, and each recipe is built around taste, time, budget, and getting the highest quality for healthy success. These are your blueprints for building a new foundation away from the comfort of the detrimental world and into the comfort of your specific course to healing. I've written this book to provide inspiration for your healthier steps forward and to put a smile into your meals. So you can once again enjoy time around the table with the ones who mean the most.

So, let's get to it!

Sincerely,

Brandon Godsey
#1 Best Selling Author: *My Simple Changes*
MySimpleChanges.com

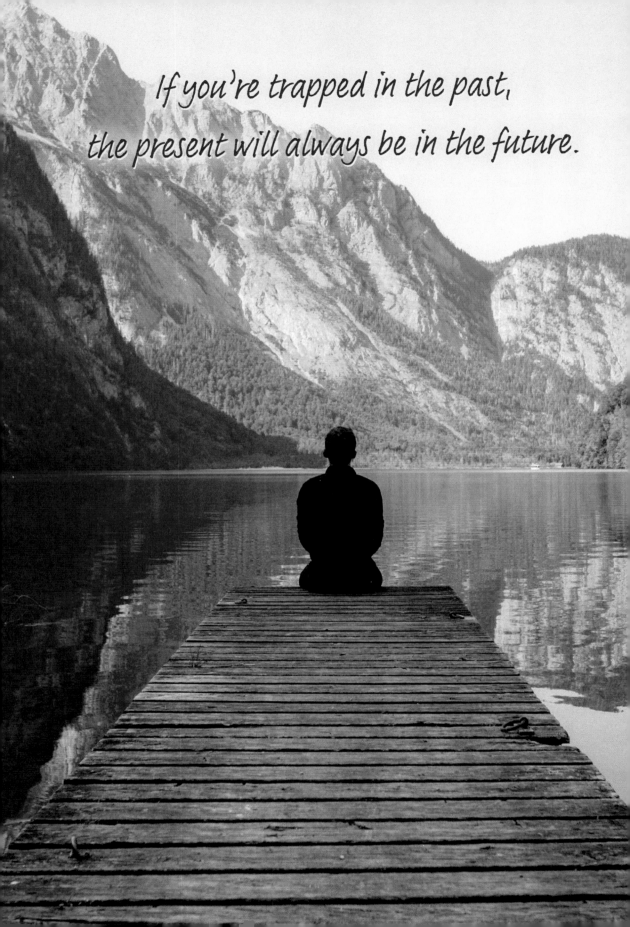

THE PHASES

PHASE 1: THE CALMING PHASE

This is when you should be on your strictest of diets to allow your body to calm, heal itself, and restore. Only you know the truth of where you are in this regard. Hold that truth and let the rest do the work.

Until you have reached a confirmed "remission," or you have been symptom-free for a few months, this phase is where you live. It's not as bad and mean as it looks. It's actually quite tasty and more available than you think. Remember, if it's hard work and it seems like you can't eat anything...
1. Everyone feels that at first... and 2. If you always see it as a challenge it'll never be a solution. See the opportunity and growth will follow.

PHASE 2: THE EXPANSION PHASE

When your system has calmed, healthy bacteria has built balance, and your system is now working to gain strength, expand the menu. Slowly. Don't overload your system because opportunity says it's now okay. Remember, it takes months or years—not days—to remission.

Balance the recipes in this phase with recipes from phase 1. An honest balance. Only you know that honesty. Don't force it.

PHASE 3: THE REINTRODUCTION PHASE

This is when the waters have calmed, the holes have plugged, the results have come in, you have built a confident routine, and your honesty can keep these dishes to a minimal, once in a while, consumption. Cherish this. Never let it go. You earned it. Celebrate by calmly holding it and acknowledging what it took to heal you to here. That's a powerful thing. The strength to stay strong. For yourself. For your health. For everything you now get to live in this, your precious life.

THE STANDARD

Rule	Reasoning
The Recipes	**YOUR NEW FOUNDATION.** Get a food allergy or sensitivity test done and identify all the other known allergies your unique life lives with. Then adjust accordingly but stay in the realm of these recipes. **NOTE: This is what the "adjust" box on various recipes offers you: your sensitivity adjustment while keeping the foundation of the healing recipes.**
Quality	**NEVER LESS** than the highest quality possible. Do you want the highest quality health? Then your standard should not be any less than the best.
Price	What you need is on sale at the right price somewhere. Stop at no cost for the highest quality. Stop telling yourself that it's expensive to be healthy. Put the money you'll save on doctors' visits and unwritten prescriptions into your food and lifestyle budget.
Organic & Non-GMO	**ALWAYS ORGANIC & non-GMO** (at the minimum). Other accredited third-party testing preferred (along with certified organic).
Variety	**DO NOT** get stuck eating the same routine of meals. **DO** get stuck in the same foundation and balancing the ingredients from there. **MEANING,** don't eat the same sweet potato bowl for breakfast twelve days straight (maybe one out of every three days, or similar)
Meat Certification	**RESEARCH.** Buy meat from heavy metal–tested or animal welfare–rated from farms you've researched that use the highest quality practices.
Portions	**ALWAYS MEASURE INGREDIENTS.** Consciously balance your day in terms of fiber, protein, carbs, saturated fat, sugar, fructose, and more. The more you know, the more control you have of your situation. These recipes are set up to be general portions. Follow the charts. Only you will know what your balance is for a meal in proportion to a day and a week of consumption. Adjust the recipes from there. **TIP:** Use smaller bowls and plates: 16-ounce bowls, 6- to 7-inch plates.
Stool Observations	**GOALS:** Pay attention to every sample. **FORMATION:** Notice the trends of what consistency comes with each day's substances, toxin exposure, and progress. **WATER & UNDIGESTED (YELLOW BILE):** Still leaking, stick to the liquids. **MUCK:** Getting better, but still not absorbing and pulling the proper nutrients. Consume probiotics and digestive enzymes! Keep them on the regular. **SOFT FORMATION:** Don't stress; this could be from a lack of antinutrient-loaded fiber. Stick to the plan. **SOLID & CRACKING:** Dehydration! You're doing okay but are not getting enough water. **PERFECT:** Not too hard, not a mush, but when the wiping leaves no residue behind… that's the goal.

PRODUCT ESSENTIALS

Product	Strategy (Always organic and non-GMO)
Avocado oil	Extra virgin
Apple cider vinegar	Raw, unfiltered with the mother 2 ingredients: apple cider vinegar and purified water
Globe Artichoke hearts	Packed in purified water
Avocado oil Olive oil	Extra virgin Unfiltered extra virgin
Chamomile flowers	Non-irradiated
Coconut aminos	Coconut nectar, sea salt
Coconut flour	1 ingredient: coconut flour
Coconut milk	Light, no guar gum (2 ingredients) Coconut and purified water
Coconut oil	Unrefined extra virgin
Coconut sugar	Unrefined
Collagen peptides	Unflavored, hydrolyzed collagen from grass-fed, pasture-raised bovine hide. *No other ingredients*
Cranberry juice	100 percent pure juice
Fermented foods (sauerkraut, kimchee, etc.)	No extra ingredients other than dill and approved whole foods from the lists. Start incorporating in Expansion Phase and observe digestive reactions. Avoid otherwise because of possible GI disruption.
Jackfruit	2 ingredients: jackfruit, purified water
Lavender flowers	Buds
Manuka honey	K-factor 16+
Maple syrup	1 ingredient: maple syrup
Microgreens	Kale, broccoli, celery, arugula *Balance by rotated variety*
Olives	Whole, unpitted olives. Observe the extra ingredients. Whole approved ingredients.
Peppermint leaves	Whole leaf
Pickles	*No calcium chloride*
Pomegranate juice	100 percent pomegranate juice
Pumpkin (canned puree)	1 ingredient: pumpkin
Salmon	Tested for heavy metals, Pacific Northwest, processed in USA, no farm raised, if canned; packed in natural juices or purified water
Sardines (or Kippers)	Cold water, wild caught, if canned; packed in natural juices
Spices	Non-irradiated
Sprouted almond flour	Sprouted and 1 ingredient: almond flour
White rice flour	Stone ground

HOME ESSENTIALS

Name	Strategy
All-purpose cleaner	Plant based, no artificial fragrances
Bar soap	Organic artisan handmade
Blender/mixer	All in one blender.
Clothing	GOTS-certified organic and vegetable dyes. (Tip: sweats, shorts, underwear, socks, t-shirts, hoodie)
Dental floss	Eco-friendly cornstarch floss picks
Dishwashing liquid	Plant based, no chlorine or artificial fragrances
Dryer balls	100 percent wool
Food storage	Glass
Laundry detergent	Plant based without dyes or fragrances
Liquid soap	Plant based, nontoxic
Pots and pans	Glass
Skillet	Cast iron
Small electronic stainless-steel scale	The best way to avoid the progress-killing trap of overconsumption is knowledge. A scale increases efficiency while decreasing chances of regression.
Smoothie blender	Bullet
Tea filter bags	Unbleached, 100 percent natural and sustainable
Toothbrush	Natural bamboo with charcoal bristles
Toothpaste	No glycerin or fluoride, organic and plant based with minimal ingredients
Utensils	Wood, silicone, stainless steel
Water bottle	Glass with bamboo top (clear borosilicate glass)

ESSENTIAL OILS

roduct	My Suggestions
il	Cedarwood, Chamomile, Cinnamon, Eucalyptus, Orange, Frankincense, Ginger, Lavender, Oregano, Peppermint, Lemon, Rose, Rose Hip Oil, Tea Tree, Ylang Ylang
arrier oil	Jojoba oil
ottles	Dark glass

SPICES

The power of spices: easily absorbable, nutrient-dense superfoods. Every spice in the method is geared toward pairing with the right ingredients to provide anti-inflammatory properties and better assist the breaking down and absorption of the rest of the meal.

Cinnamon	Sage
Dill	Tarragon
Ginger, ground	Thyme
Oregano	Turmeric, ground
Rosemary	

SUPPLEMENTS

Name	My Dosage Strategy
Collagen peptides	1 scoop per sitting (up to 2 scoops a day, but not every day)
Digestive enzyme	1 capsule 20 to 30 minutes before a meal, per day (maybe 2 a day, but not every day)
Oil of oregano (liquid)	3 ingredients: oregano, grain alcohol, water
Probiotics	Only probiotic strains specific to building in bowels & only probiotics; no other ingredients
Turmeric pills	2 ingredients: black pepper and turmeric 1 to 3 pills a day (but not every day)
Vitamin D	Liquid and olive oil only

MY SIMPLE FOODS LISTS

Fall back on these lists when you need to adjust—
but can't remember what to adjust to!

Inflammation-Healing Foods

Very Important	
Water (purified, 64 to 80 ounces per day)	
Fruits	
Blueberries	Raspberries
Cherries	Strawberries
Oranges	Tangerines
Pineapple	
Vegetables	
Any leafy green	Chard
Artichokes	Collard Greens
Arugula	Garlic
Avocados	Kale
Beets	Leeks
Bok choy	Maca
Broccoli	Mushrooms
Brussels sprouts	Olives
Cabbage	Onions
Carrots	Spinach
Celery	Sweet potatoes (all varieties)
Cauliflower	
Oils	
Avocado	Olive
Coconut	

Inflammation-Triggering Foods

Alcohol (all varieties)	Processed foods
Chicken	Red meat (low quality/high fat/ excessive amounts)
Dairy	Salt
Fried foods	Soda
Fruit juices	Sugar-sweetened drink
High glycemic–index foods (sugar and grains)	Vegetable oils (corn, safflower/ sunflower, soybean, peanut, cottonseed)
Margarine	

High-Fiber Foods

erving Size	Daily Goal
cup	25 to 50 grams (spread out)

ote: General rule of thumb- no seeds, no skins. Until fully healed and tolerated.

Vegetables

ame	Fiber per serving	Preparation
corn squash	9 grams	Baked cubes
rtichoke hearts	9.6 grams	Boiled
sparagus	4 grams	Baked or sautéed
roccoli	5.5 grams	Steamed
russels sprouts	4 grams	Steamed
utternut squash	7 grams	Baked cubes
auliflower	5 grams	Steamed
ollard greens	5 grams	Sautéed
emp seeds (per ounce)	10 grams	Shelled, raw
ale	3 grams	Sautéed
ustard greens	5 grams	Sautéed
kra	4 grams	Steamed
arsnips	7 grams	Raw
umpkin	8 grams	Baked cubes
urple sweet potato	5 grams	Baked cubes
pinach	4 grams	Sautéed
weet potato	4 grams	Baked cubes
wiss chard	4 grams	Sautéed

Fruits

ame	Fiber per serving	Preparation
vocado	3.5 grams	¼ medium avocado
aspberries	8 grams	Whole
range	4.5 grams	Pieces
ananas	3.5 grams	7- to 8-inch medium
omegranate	6 grams	Seeds
uava	9 grams	Cubes
ackfruit	3 grams	Canned in water

FODMAP FOODS
Fermentable Oligo-, Di, Monosaccharides And Polyols

FODMAP foods are a collection of short-chain carbohydrates found in many common foods that result in an increased volume of liquid and gas in the small and large intestine, causing further disruptions and irritation.

Low-FODMAP Foods to Consume

Vegetables	
Bamboo shoots	Ginger
Bok choi	Kale
Carrots	Lettuce
Chives	Olives
Cucumber	Turnips
Fruits	
Bananas	Limes
Blueberries	Oranges
Lemon	Strawberries
Other	
All meats	Ginger tea
Coconut milk (no guar gum)	Purified water
Cranberry juice	

High-FODMAP Foods to Avoid

Vegetables	
Artichokes	Celery
Asparagus	Garlic
Brussels sprouts	Leeks
Cabbage	Mushrooms
Fruits	
Apricots	Nectarines
Cherries	Peaches
Coconut water	Plums
Dried fruit	Prunes
Fruit juices	

Fructose-Friendly Foods

Excess fructose gets stuck in the gut and grows problematic bacteria, which can lead to SIBO, leaky gut, and malabsorption. Digestive disorders mean fewer cells in the gut to absorb fructose, making the problem even more sensitive. Healthy GI tracts should be limited to 20 to 35 grams of fructose daily. Unhealthy GI tracts should limit to virtually none.

Vegetables		Fruits	
Beets	Mushrooms	Apricot	Lime
Carrot	Okra	Avocado	Nectarine
Celery	Radish	Banana	Peach
Cucumber	Spinach	Blueberries	Pineapple
Iceberg Lettuce	Sweet Potato	Cranberries	Plum
		Fig, fresh	Raspberries
		Grapefruit	Rhubarb
		Jackfruit	Sour Cherries
		Lemon	

High-Protein Foods

Serving	Daily Goal
cup, or 4 ounces when listed	30% to 50% body weight, or 10% of daily calorie intake

Vegetables

Name	Protein per serving	Preparation
Artichoke	4 grams	Steamed
Arugula	3 grams	Raw
Asparagus	3 grams	Lightly sautéed
Bamboo shoots	4 grams	½-inch slices, raw
Beet greens	3.5 grams	Sautéed
Broccoli	4 grams	Steamed
Brussels sprouts	4.5 grams	Steamed
Butternut squash	2 grams	Roasted
Cauliflower, chopped	2 grams	Steamed
Collard greens	5 grams	Sautéed
Garlic	1 gram	Raw
Kale	2.5 grams	Sautéed
Leeks	4 grams	Raw
Portabella mushrooms	4 grams	Grilled
Seaweed	2 grams	Raw
Shitake mushrooms	3.5 grams	Sautéed
Spinach	5 grams	Steamed
Vine leaf	4.5 grams	Steamed
White mushrooms	3.5 grams	Sautéed

Fruits

Name	Protein per serving	Preparation
Apricots	2.2 grams	Sliced
Apricots	2.2g	Sliced
Avocado	3 grams	Sliced, mashed
Bananas	1.3 grams	Sliced
Blackberries	2 grams	Whole
Kiwifruit	2.1 grams	Sliced
Oranges	2 grams	Sliced
Peaches	1.5 grams	Sliced
Raspberries	1.5 grams	Whole

Broth

Name	Protein per serving	Serving Size
Beef bone broth	9 grams	1 cup
Chicken bone broth	9 grams	1 cup
Turkey bone broth	9 grams	1 cup

Meats/Seafood

Source	Protein per serving
Beef liver	31 grams
Beef, top round	25 grams
Bison	24 grams
Lamb	25 grams
Oysters	8 grams
Pork loin	25 grams
Salmon	28 grams
Sardines	23 grams
Turkey breast (baked)	30 grams

MEATS

The goal is to phase meat out as healing progresses; sprouted proteins can be reincorporated in the Reintroduction phase.

All Phases	
(foundation for all three)	
Source	**Serving Size**
Beef, top round	4 to 6 ounces
Bone Broth	8 ounces
Salmon	4 to 6 ounces
Turkey	4 to 6 ounces
Expansion Phase	
("once in a while" after healing)	
Source	**Serving Size**
Beef liver	4 ounces
Bison	4 ounces
Lamb	4 ounces
Sardines or Kippers	6 ounces
Reintroduction Phase	
(a rarity in the healthiest of times)	
Source	**Serving Size**
Oysters	4 to 6 shells
Pork loin	4 ounces
Tuna	6 ounces

DIGESTION STRETCHES

Do these stretches while lying on your back, and in this order.
Hold all poses for 15 to 30 seconds, at minimum.

1. Bound angle pose	6. Lying twist to left	11. Morning stretch	16. Happy Baby pose
2. Knees to chest pose	7. Knees to chest	12. Figure four pose (left foot)	17. Knees to chest
3. Lying twist to right	8. Morning stretch pose	13. Morning stretch	18. Bridge pose
4. Morning stretch pose	9. Knees to chest	14. Bound angle pose	19. Broad angle pose
5. Knees to chest	10. Figure four pose (right foot)	15. Morning stretch	NOT ON BACK: 10 to 20 Cat/Cow poses

PREPARING VEGETABLES

Start incorporating raw in the Expansion Phase.
For all phases, stick mainly to steamed, roasted, or sautéed

Steamed

Vegetable	Prep	Steaming Time (minutes)
Acorn squash	Cut into 1-inch cubes	10 to 12
Asparagus	Whole (tough ends snapped off)	9 to 12
Beets	Cut into 1-inch cubes	30 to 45
Broccoli	Cut into florets	5 to 8
Brussels sprouts	Bases trimmed, cut in half	10 to 14
Butternut squash	Cut into 1-inch cubes	10
Carrots	Cut into 3-inch pieces	8 to 10
Cauliflower	Cut into florets	8 to 10
Onions	Cut into 3-inch strings	10
Sweet potatoes	Cut into 1-inch cubes	10 to 12

Roasted

Vegetable	Prep	Baking Time, Temp
Acorn squash	Cut in half; discard seeds and strings; lightly oil cut surfaces	45 minutes, 375°
Asparagus	Whole; tough ends snapped off	25 minutes, 350°
Beets	Whole (wrapped in foil)	45 minutes, 375° degrees
Broccoli	Cut into 1- to 2-inch florets	20 minutes, 375°
Brussels sprouts	Bases trimmed; cut in half	25 minutes, 350°
Butternut squash	Cut in half; discard seeds and strings; lightly oil cut surfaces	45 minutes, 375°
Carrots	Cut in half lengthwise then into 3-inch pieces	20 minutes, 375°
Cauliflower	Cut into 1- to 2-inch florets	20 minutes, 375°
Celery	Cut into ½-inch dice	20 minutes, 375°
Mushrooms	Cut in half	25 minutes, 350°
Onions	Cut into 3-inch strings	20 minutes, 375°
Sweet potatoes	Cut into 1-inch cubes or fries	45 minutes, 375°
Spaghetti squash	Cut in half; discard seeds and strings; lightly oil cut surfaces	50 minutes, 375°

A DAY IN THE CHANGES

This is the foundation day. All subsequent days build and adjust from here. Mold around your current condition and the day's requirements, but stick to the plan.

Order	Suggestion	Explanation
1	Welcome to the day	Don't even think about that device! Set the tone of the day with calming ease and avoid electronics for the first hour of the day.
2	Brush teeth	Bamboo toothbrush & fluoride-free toothpaste
3	Digestive stretches	In bed or on a yoga mat
4	Warm purified or alkaline water	8 to 12 ounces (optional: collagen peptides, lemon/lime juice, ACV or oregano oil)
5	Exercise	30 to 45 minutes mild exercise (don't overdo it!).
6	Probiotic &/or digestive enzyme	20 to 30 minutes before meal Probiotic: 5 billion (to start; expand as digestive comfort grows acceptance) Digestive enzyme: 1 full-spectrum pill
7	**Meal #1**	Medium in size and heaviness
8	Tea, purified or alkaline water (room temperature)	8 to 12 ounces 1-2 hours after meal
9	Deep stretching, meditation, and/or sleep	Do what your body calls for!
10	Probiotic & digestive enzyme	20 to 30 minutes before meal After baseline grows, incorporate second dose (starting with 5 billion). 8 to 12 ounces water
11	**Meal #2**	3 to 5 hours after meal #1 Largest meal of the day, usually involving the heaviest foods to digest.
12	Water	8 to 12 ounces 45 to 60 minutes after meal
13	Stretch, yoga, meditation or sleep	Whatever your body is calling for. Balance your day for your condition.
14	**Meal #3**	Small and light. (example: 8 ounce smoothie or piece of fruit)
15	Digestive enzyme	Optional. Don't overdo it but do it!! 1-2 pills a day and not every day. (20-30 minutes before meal)
16	**Meal #4**	Small and light. (Example: 8 to 12 ounces of broth with veggies and a small amount of protein) & at least 2-4 hours before bed.
17	Warm water or tea	8 to 12 ounces 1 hour, or so, before bed (optional: lemon or lime juice)
18	Brush teeth	Bamboo toothbrush & fluoride-free toothpaste
19	Digestion stretches and meditation	Usually in bed!! Balance your meditation throughout the day.
20	Sleep	As long as your body is calling for it. Don't cut off repairs in progress. Aim for at least 7 hours sleep a night.
21	Repeat	Until the situation has calmed (weeks to months). Listen to your body, and smile.

THE
CALMING
PHASE

Let go of what once was.
Now is the time to be the change.

THE CALMING PHASE

These recipes are the foundation and are dedicated for the times when your body is at its highest degree of sensitivity and inflammation. Or when expansion happens a little too fast and you need to take a step back to your foundation. Or when the inevitable, out-of-our-control happens and regression arrives. Wherever you are, these are the recipes and ingredients that offer the best chances for relief. With trust, commitment, and patience, these ingredients and recipes remain the pillars for keeping your growth looking forward.

Only you will know the truth to this question: "Am I ready to move on to the next phase?" When you believe it to be true, then move your smiles to the expansion phase and congratulate yourself with a celebration. But don't ever forget, the calming phase makes up the majority of your days. Everything else balances minimally and accordingly.

While in this phase, take the time to allow your body to calm and repair, incorporating supplements, stress routines, extremely light workouts, breathing, and meditation into your balanced day of eating.

Forget about the norms. Forget about time. Forget about that line to stand in. Forget about that deadline to cram in. Forget everything but the most important thing to your life: your health. Without it, you have nothing. With it, you give your world everything.

NOTES:

- *Yoga and meditation are essential during this phase, as well as learning to breathe, stretching, and doing digestive twists. Be as gentle on your body as possible during this phase. This applies to consumption, exercise, stress, rest, and avoiding over-supplementation. Limit exercise to non-strenuous walks that are no more than two to five miles, and remain conscious of your exertion. Too much will create more stress than your gastrointestinal tract can handle and will cause disruptions and inflammation.*

- *Probiotics- Slowly increase from 5-400 billion, depending on comfort.*

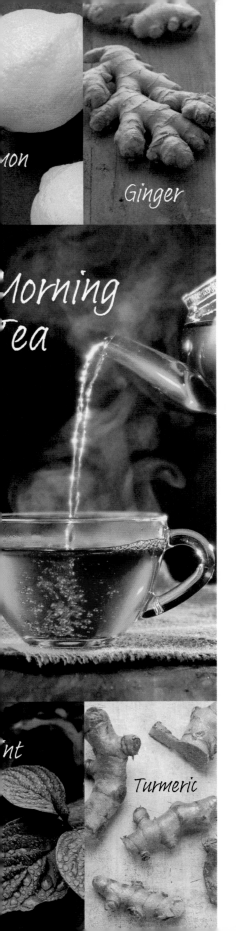

TEA

Lemon
Ingredients

8 to 12 ounces purified water

Juice of ¼ to ½ medium lemon,
or 1 tablespoon unpasteurized
apple cider vinegar

1 scoop collagen peptides

½ teaspoon ground cinnamon

Ginger
Ingredients

2 cups purified water
(or alkaline)

1 tablespoon minced peeled
fresh ginger

1 slice lemon

½ teaspoon ground cinnamon

Mint
Ingredients

2 to 3 cups purified water

4 to 6 fresh peppermint leaves

½ teaspoon ground cinnamon

Turmeric
Ingredients

12 ounces purified water

1 tablespoon minced
fresh turmeric root

1 teaspoon ground cinnamon

1 slice lemon

Instructions

Warm purified water until just before it boils, or simmer the
ginger for 10 minutes.

Combine the solid ingredients in an unbleached tea bag (if
applicable) and squeeze the liquid ingredients into the water.

Enjoy that fresh start!

*Deep Breaths.. 4 beats in..
2 beats hold.. 5 beats out.. repeat.*

*The caffeine and antinutrients in coffee beans can
irritate your gut lining, cause intestinal contractions,
and ultimately disrupt digestion. Answer? Tea or
warm water with lemon.*

TURKEY BONE BROTH

Daily 3:1
liquid to solid ratio until
the system throbbing calms

Ingredients

1 gallon purified water

Bones from Oven-Roasted Turkey Breast (page 45)

2 medium to large carrots, chopped into ¼-inch rounds

4 celery stalks, chopped into ¼-inch rounds

2 tablespoons unpasteurized apple cider vinegar

1 teaspoon pink Himalayan sea salt

1 sprig fresh thyme

1 sprig fresh rosemary

This is your meal. Make notes. Find your ingredient balance.

Instructions

Combine all the ingredients in a large pot over high heat and bring to a boil.

Cover the pot and reduce the heat to low.

Simmer for at least 12 hours and up to 24 hours without stirring (the longer the better).

Strain and store the broth for 7 to 10 days.

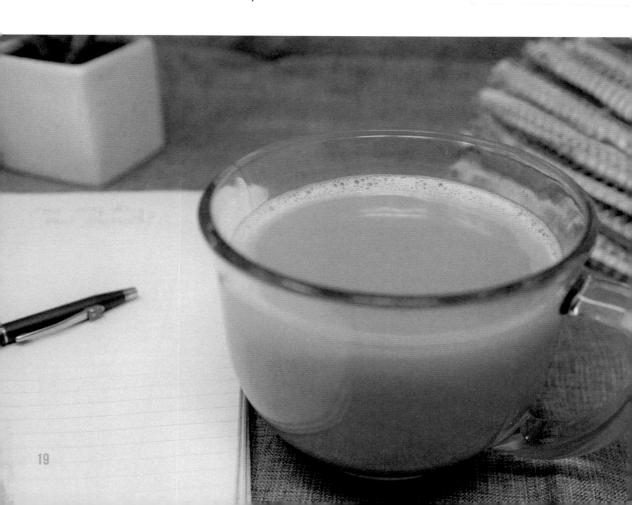

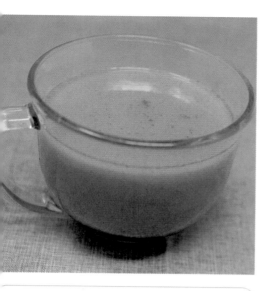

BEEF BONE BROTH

Ingredients

1 gallon purified water

3 to 5 pounds beef bones

2 medium to large carrots

4 celery stalks

2 tablespoons apple cider vinegar

1 teaspoon pink Himalayan sea salt

1 sprig fresh rosemary

6 stems fresh parsley

Chop through these recipes. Freeze the trimmings. Build the collection, make broth, let cool, and freeze as cubes.
Uses: *smoothies, starter liquid, sipping.*

Instructions

Combine all the ingredients in a large pot over high heat and bring to a boil.

Cover the pot and reduce the heat to low.

Simmer for at least 12 hours and up to 24 hours without stirring (the longer the better).

VEGGIE STOCK CUBES

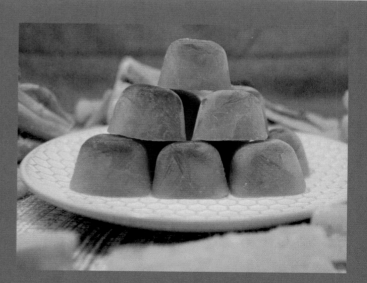

Ingredients

vegetable trimmings

purified water

Instructions

When preparing other meals, save the vegetable and herb stems, trimmings, and peels.

Keep them in a freezer-safe glass storage container, adding more until the container is full.

Combine the trimmings and water in a large pot over high heat, and bring to a boil.

Cover the pot, reduce the heat to low, and simmer for 2 to 3 hours.

Strain. Let cool and freeze in ice cube trays.

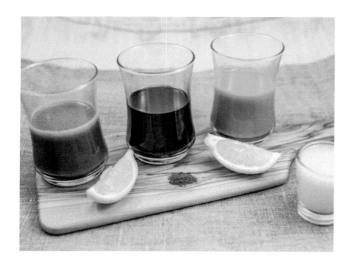

ABSORPTION BLEND

Ingredients

2 ounces (¼ cup) juiced fresh ginger

1½ ounces (1 shot) kale juice

1½ ounces (1 shot) ginger juice

3 ounces (2 shots) pomegranate juice

3 ounces (2 shots) carrot juice

¼ juiced lemon

1 teaspoon ground cinnamon

1 teaspoon turmeric powder or grated fresh

Instructions

Combine all the ingredients in a glass bottle and shake for 1 minute.

Pour into a glass over purified ice.

JUICY REJUVENATION

Ingredients

2 ounces (¼ cup) celery juice

2 ounces (¼ cup) orange juice

2 ounces (¼ cup) beet juice

2 ounces (¼ cup) kale juice

Juice of ¼ lime

1 teaspoon ground cinnamon

1 teaspoon ground turmeric

Instructions

Combine all the ingredients in a glass bottle and shake for 1 minute.

Pour into a glass over purified ice.

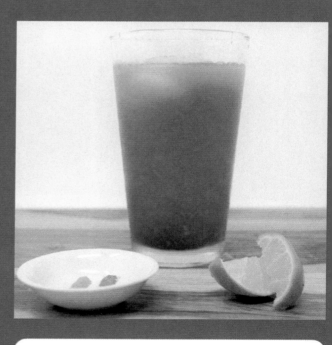

Blending pre-digest's the food. Allowing fruits to digest easier with healthy fats and protein.

CREAMBERRY SMOOTHIE

Ingredients

- 1 cup frozen blueberries
- 1 cup pressed kale
- 1 inch minced peeled fresh ginger
- 1 medium carrot
- 1 cup Bone Broth (page 19)
- 3 or 4 cubes purified ice
- 1 teaspoon ground cinnamon
- 1 teaspoon turmeric powder (or grated fresh)
- 1 tablespoon maple syrup

Instructions

Combine all the ingredients in a smoothie maker or blender. Blend until creamy smooth.

Patience

Persistence

Perseverance

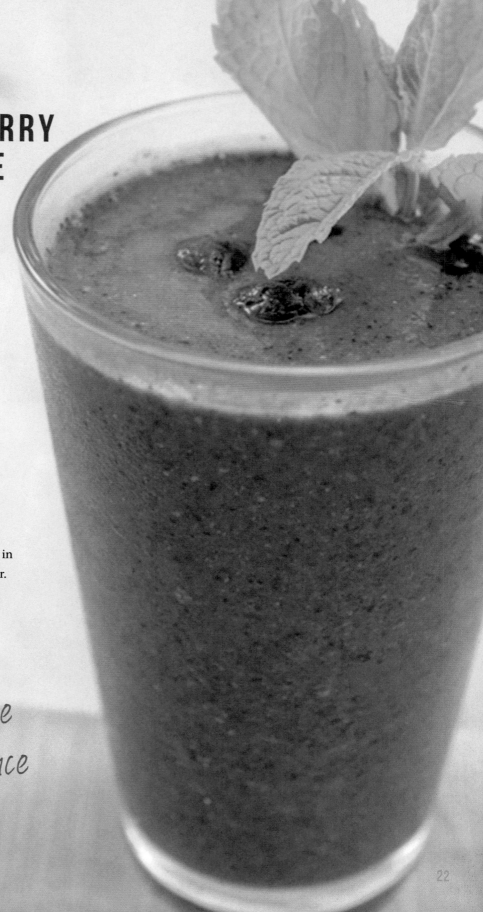

THE CLASSIC

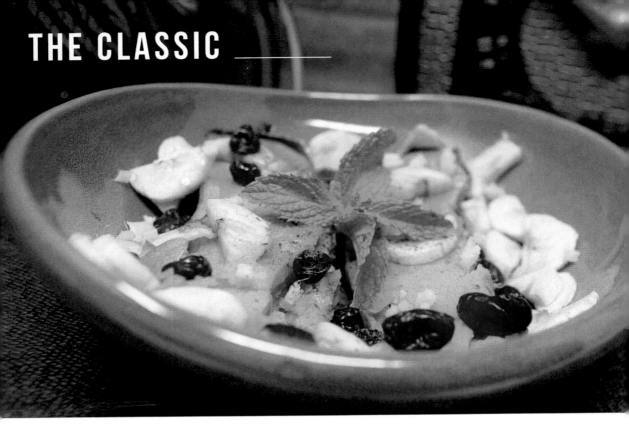

Ingredients

1 medium sweet potato, cubed (½ to 2/3 cup)

1 tablespoon purified water

1 scoop collagen peptides

Cranberry sauce

½ medium green banana or ½ cup raspberries

1 teaspoon ground cinnamon

1 teaspoon turmeric powder

1 teaspoon minced peeled fresh ginger

1 teaspoon coconut oil

½ tablespoon maple syrup

Optional

4 ounces turkey breast

¼ cup microgreens

Instructions

Bake the sweet potato at 375° for roughly 30 minutes or until easily pierced with a fork.

In a small bowl, combine the water and collagen peptides. Allow to dissolve.

In a bowl, fan open the sweet potato and top with the peptides and remaining ingredients.

CRANBERRY SAUCE

Ingredients

¼ cup frozen cranberries

2 tablespoons purified water

2 teaspoons minced peeled fresh ginger

1 teaspoon manuka honey

Instructions

Combine all the ingredients in a small saucepan over medium heat.

Simmer gently until the liquid has evaporated and the cranberries have cracked, 4 to 5 minutes.

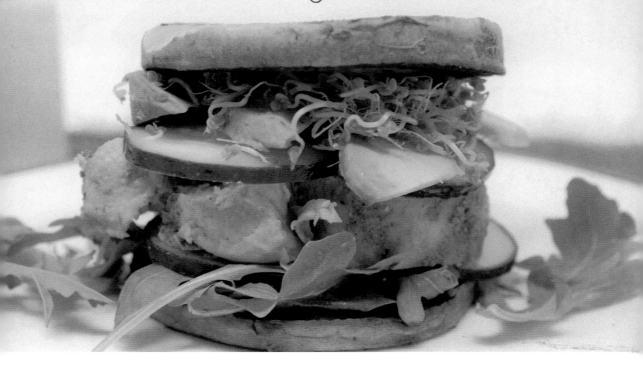

YAM-BAM BREAKFAST SANDWICH

Ingredients

1 fat yam

½ tablespoon coconut oil

1 teaspoon pink Himalayan sea salt

¼ cup pressed fresh arugula

½ medium avocado

Pinch broccoli sprouts or microgreens

3 or 4 peeled cucumbers, thinly sliced and seeds removed

Sliced baked turkey (page 45)

Fruits: Eaten alone and on an empty stomach or halve the serving and only consume low-sugar options to eliminate fermenting (feeding) bad bacteria in the gut.

Optional

Teeth Mark's cheese (page 80) (**Note:** this will reclassify the recipe as a Reintroduction Phase recipe)

Instructions

Thoroughly wash the yam. Cut it into 1/3- to ½-inch-thick rounds.

In a medium saucepan on medium heat, warm the coconut oil.

Add the yam rounds and cook, undisturbed, for 3 to 4 minutes.

Flip them and cook for another 2 to 3 minutes.

On a plate, stack the remaining ingredients on top of one yam round and cover with another to complete your sandwich. Extra rounds can be stored for future sandwiches.

HASH IT OUT BOWL

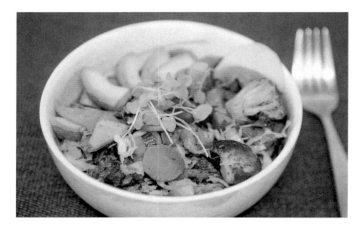

Instructions

In a cast iron skillet on medium heat, warm the olive oil.

Strain, rinse, and dry the sweet potato cubes.

Add the sweet potatoes to the skillet and cook, stirring occasionally, for 7 to 10 minutes or until slightly soft and lightly golden brown.

Add the remaining ingredients and cook for 3 to 4 minutes, continuing to stir. Remove from the heat, stir, and serve with your desired toppings.

Ingredients

1 tablespoon olive oil

1 medium sweet potato, chopped into ¼- to ½-inch cubes and soaked for at least 1 hour in purified water and a splash of apple cider vinegar

½ cup finely chopped leek

½ cup roughly chopped broccoli

1 cup purple kale

¼ cup shaved Brussels sprouts

½ cup chopped carrots (¼-inch rounds)

1 celery stalk, chopped

1 teaspoon chopped fresh sage

1 teaspoon dried rosemary

Ground turmeric

1 tablespoon coconut aminos

Juice of ½ lemon

Toppings

Microgreens

½ sliced avocado

¼ cup sprouted black beans, soaked and cooked (optional) (note: This addition will reclassify the recipe to the Reintroduction Phase

Turkey breast (optional)

AVOCADO MAYO

Ingredients

1 medium avocado

½ cup melted coconut butter

½ cup purified water

½ cup olive oil

2 tablespoons lemon juice

1 teaspoon ground turmeric

1 tablespoon maple syrup

1 teaspoon coconut aminos

Instructions

Combine all the ingredients in a blender or food processor and blend until thickened, 2 to 3 minutes.

Strain into a glass jar and store in the refrigerator.

Note: If the mayo is too dry, add more olive oil.

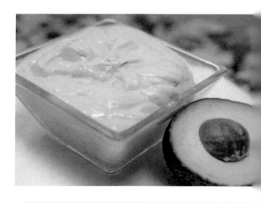

Be conscious of daily saturated fat content. Although coconut has several beneficial qualities, it is also high in saturated fats. Which cause disruptions along the gastrointestinal tract.

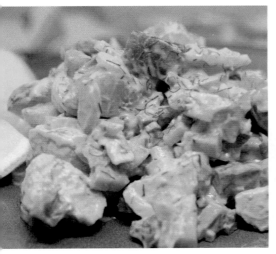
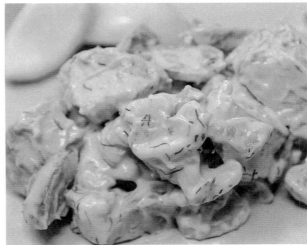

URKEY
ALAD

gredients
p chopped Oven-Roasted Turkey Breast
ge 45)
elery stalk, diced
arrot, diced
allion, sliced
blespoons finely chopped leek
edium roasted golden beet, chopped
ge 14)
easpoon minced fresh dill
easpoon ground turmeric
easpoon dried sage
up Avocado Mayo (page 25) *add more if
xture is too dry

structions
mbine the turkey, vegetables, herbs, and
ces in a bowl.
d the avocado mayo and gently stir until
roughly combined.
te: You can trade out the turkey breast for
mon or a sweet potato.

SWEET POTATO
SALAD

Ingredients
*Same as turkey salad, but substitute the turkey with
1 medium baked sweet potato, diced (page 14)
1 medium roasted beet, diced (page 14)

Instructions
Preheat the oven to 400°.
Wash, scrub, and dry the sweet potato and beets.
Bake for 30 to 45 minutes until fork tender
(avoid overcooking… think "a little crunchy").
While allowing the sweet potato and beets to
completely cool (tip: stick them in the refrigerator),
chop the necessary ingredients.
Dice the cooled sweet potato and beets.
Combine in a large glass bowl with
the remaining ingredients.
Gently stir until thoroughly combined.

*This recipe, and all meals, are your
serving size. If the ingredients don't
specify amounts, you'll know the
blend you need.*

VEGGIELICIOUSNESS

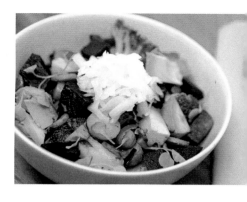

Ingredients
Thinly sliced collard greens
Thinly sliced leek (green parts only)
Rainbow-colored carrots, chopped
Broccoli florets
Diced beets
Unpitted black olives
Diced peeled cucumber, seeds removed
1 tablespoon minced peeled fresh ginger
Juice of 1 lime
1 teaspoon coconut aminos
1 teaspoon ground turmeric
1 tablespoon oil
Pinch dried tarragon

Toppings
Microgreens
Sauerkraut
Avocado slices

Instructions
In a medium pan on medium heat, warm the avocado oil. Combine all the ingredients (except for the toppings) in the pan and sauté for 3 to 5 minutes. Transfer to a bowl and top with the microgreens, sauerkraut, and avocado.

Reach.
Achieve.
Reach again.

All ~~good~~ bad things come to an end.

SPAGHETTI WRAP

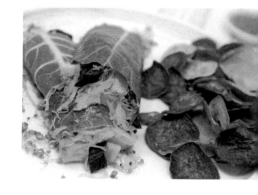

Ingredients
½ cup diced roasted beet (page 14)
½ cup baked spaghetti squash (page 14)
1 tablespoon olive oil
¼ avocado, sliced
¼ cup sauerkraut
½ inch peeled cucumber, chopped and seeds removed
½ scallion, sliced
Pinch broccoli sprouts
1 teaspoon coconut aminos
Lemon juice
Sweet Ginger Sauce (page 49)
Collard greens leaves, washed, dried, and cut to desired size

Instructions
Combine the beet, squash, avocado, sauerkraut, cucumber, scallion and sprouts in a bowl. Sprinkle with the coconut aminos, lemon juice and sweet ginger sauce to taste, and toss.
Fill the collard greens leaves with the mixture and roll to your desired size.

Exercising in the morning improves production of melatonin. Helping to fight cancer development and regulate digestion.

SALAD ON-THE-RUN
W/LEMON OIL DRESSING

Ingredients

4 to 6 unpitted black olives

1 cup arugula

½ medium carrot, sliced

¼ avocado, diced

¼ cup broccoli sprouts

¼ cup diced peeled cucumber, seeds removed

¼ cup diced roasted beets

2 tablespoons sauerkraut

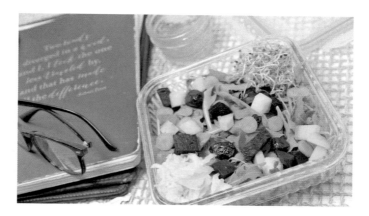

Optional

4 to 6 ounces Oven-Roasted Turkey Breast (page 45)

Instructions

Pit the olives.

Toss all the ingredients together and store in a glass container.

Place the container in a bag with a small ice pack.

LEMON OIL DRESSING

Ingredients

1 tablespoon lemon juice

1 tablespoon olive oil

1 teaspoon minced peeled fresh ginger

1 teaspoon ground turmeric

Instructions

In a small glass bottle, combine all the ingredients and shake.

Drizzle the dressing on the salad and toss in a sealed glass to-go container to evenly combine.

LIGHT VINAIGRETTE

Ingredients

½ cup olive oil

1 tablespoon apple cider vinegar

1 tablespoon lemon juice

½ teaspoon pink Himalayan sea salt

1½ teaspoons manuka honey (or maple syrup)

Instructions

Combine all the ingredients into a glass jar and shake until well combined.

Drizzle onto your food, being conscious of the amount you use.

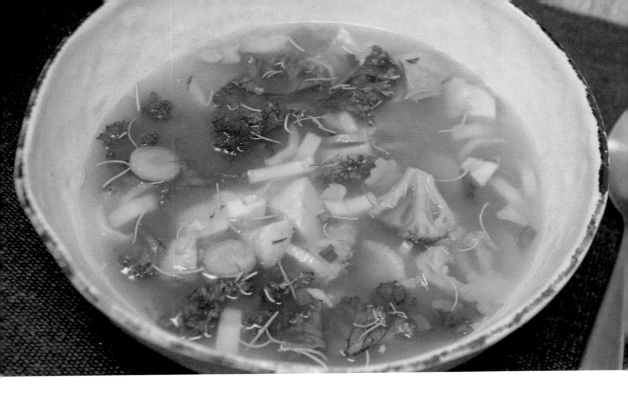

VEGETABLE SOUP

Every day you want to quit.
Then you realize, you face these
adversities because you have yet to.

Ingredients

2 cups Bone Broth (page 19)
½ medium carrot, sliced
½ medium celery stalk, sliced
½ cup roughly chopped broccoli florets
½ cup (1-inch strips) purple kale
1 tablespoon apple cider vinegar
½ teaspoon pink Himalayan sea salt
1 sprig fresh rosemary
1 gallon purified water

Toppings

½ medium avocado
1 scallion

Optional

4 ounces ground turkey or steak

Instructions

In a large pot over high heat, combine all the ingredients
except for the toppings and bring to a boil.
Cover the pot and reduce the heat to low. Simmer for 1 hour.
Gently mix the soup ingredients and serve in a bowl topped
with the scallion and avocado.

Cut the portion in half. Eat slower. Enjoy the
flavor. Wait twenty minutes. Then decide on
more, or not. Allow digestion time to alert the
brain about fullness.

Goal: 3-5 servings of greens a day. Variety,
blend, and spaced out.

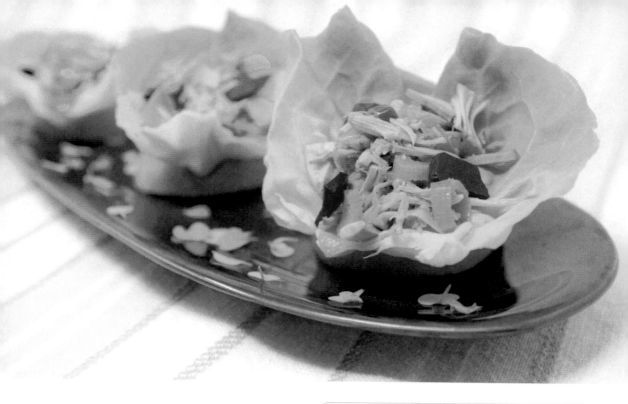

JACKFRUIT TACOS

These tacos also pair well with Savory Plantain Chips (page 33) or dipped in Sweet Ginger Sauce (page 49).

Ingredients

1 can jackfruit (no brine), drained

¼ cup thinly sliced leeks

¼ cup minced celery

¼ cup minced carrots

1 teaspoon olive oil

1 cup Bone Broth (page 19)

1 tablespoon coconut aminos

2 teaspoons ground turmeric

1 inch peeled fresh ginger, minced

1 tablespoon dried rosemary

1 teaspoon dried sage

3 to 5 butter lettuce leaves

¼ avocado

½ roasted beet, thinly sliced (page 14)

¼ cup microgreens

Instructions

Gently break apart the jackfruit with a fork.

In a large sauté pan over medium-low heat, combine the jackfruit with the leeks, mushrooms, celery, carrots, olive oil, bone broth, coconut aminos, turmeric, ginger, rosemary, and sage.

Simmer until the liquids have cooked off, 6 to 10 minutes, while using a spatula or fork to gently mix and break up the jackfruit even more as it cooks.

Line a plate with your desired number of lettuce cups and fill with the jackfruit mixture.

Top with the avocado, beet, and microgreens.

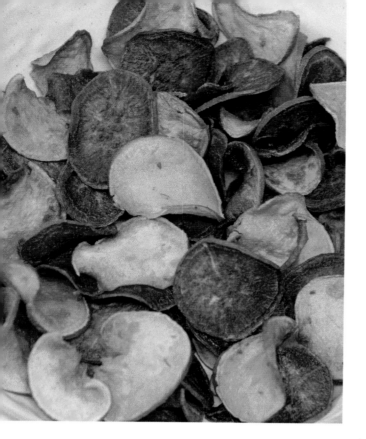

SWEET TATER CHIPPIES

Ingredients

1 medium to large sweet potato
(purple, jewel, white, yam, etc.)
1 cup coconut oil, or avocado oil
1 teaspoon pink Himalayan sea salt

Instructions

Use a mandolin or knife to slice the sweet pota
into thin "chips."
Heat a sauté pan on medium-high heat and po
in enough oil to cover the slices.
Add the sweet potato slices to the oil a few at a
time to prevent them from sticking together.
Fry until lightly golden brown, 5 to 7 minutes.
Scoop the cooked tater chips onto a paper tow
lined plate and immediately toss with the salt.

CRISPY CARROT FRIES

Ingredients

3 to 5 medium multicolored carrots,
cut into thin "fries"
1 tablespoon olive oil
½ teaspoon pink Himalayan sea salt

Instructions

Preheat the oven to 400°. Line a baking sheet
with parchment paper.
In a large bowl, toss the carrots with the oil
and sprinkle with the salt.
Spread the fries out in a single layer on the
baking sheet and bake for 15 to 20 minutes.
When the fries reach your desired crispiness,
remove them from the oven and let cool.
Serve as a side, with a dip, or as a snack.

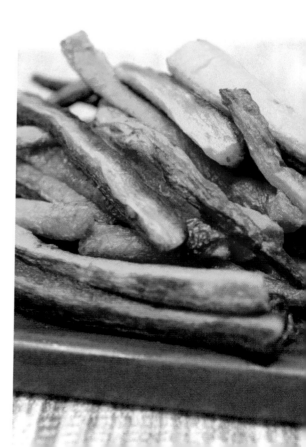

"I feel good now, one time won't hurt."

Yes it will. You just may not feel it.

CRUNCH CHIPS

Ingredients

2 cups roughly chopped kale
1 tablespoon olive oil
1 teaspoon pink Himalayan sea salt

Instructions

Preheat the oven to 325°. Line a baking sheet with parchment paper.
Dump the kale onto the parchment paper. Drizzle with the oil and gently toss until evenly coated.
Spread the kale out into a thin layer and sprinkle evenly with the salt.
Bake for 15 to 30 minutes or until the kale bakes to your desired crispiness.

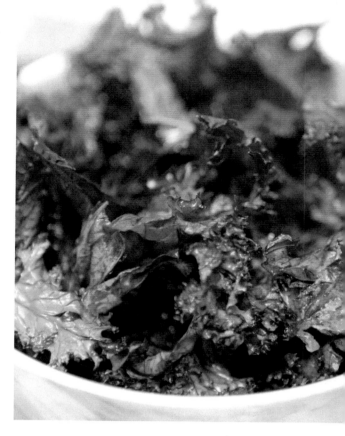

BEET CHIPS

Ingredients

½ to 1 cup avocado oil, or coconut oil
1 medium golden beet, very thinly sliced
1 medium red beet, very thinly sliced
Pinch pink Himalayan sea salt

Instructions

Into a small pot on just above medium heat, pour enough oil to cover the chips.
Working in batches, add the beets and slowly fry until slightly golden, turning every so often.
Scoop the cooked chips onto a paper towel–lined plate and immediately toss with the salt.

BAKED BRUSSELS SPROUTS

Ingredients

2 cups halved Brussels sprouts
2 tablespoons olive oil
1 scallion, chopped
Pinch pink Himalayan sea salt

Instructions

Preheat the oven to 400°. Line a baking sheet with tin foil.
Combine the sprouts and oil in a bowl, then spread out on the baking sheet.
Bake for 10 minutes. Toss, spread out, and cook for another 10 minutes.
Transfer to a bowl and top with the scallion.

GUACAMOLE

Ingredients

1 medium avocado

½ scallion, thinly sliced

1 tablespoon finely chopped leeks

Juice of ½ lime

Pinch ground turmeric

Pinch pink Himalayan sea salt

1 teaspoon coconut aminos

Dippers

1 medium carrot,
cut into 2- to
3-inch strips

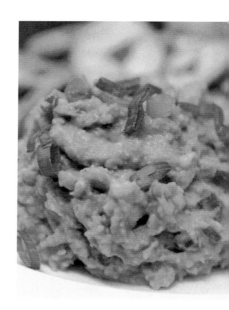

Instructions

Mash the avocado.

Add the scallion, leeks, turmeric, salt, and coconut aminos and mix thoroughly.

Pour in the lime juice and gently mix until well combined.

Transfer the guacamole to a plate or bowl and serve with the cucumber and carrot.

SAVORY PLANTAIN CHIPS

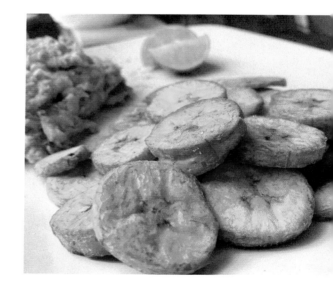

Ingredients

1 medium green plantain

1 cup coconut oil

2 teaspoons pink Himalayan sea salt

Instructions

Cut off the ends of the plantains and peel the outer shell off, just as you would a banana.

Use a mandolin or knife to slice the plantains into thin "chips."

Heat a sauté pan on medium-high heat and pour in enough coconut oil to cover the chips.

Add the plantain slices to the oil a few at a time to prevent them sticking together.

Fry until lightly golden brown, roughly 5 minutes.

Scoop the cooked chips onto a paper towel–lined plate and immediately sprinkle with the salt. (It's much easier to have a friendly salt assistant!)

CARROT PUREE

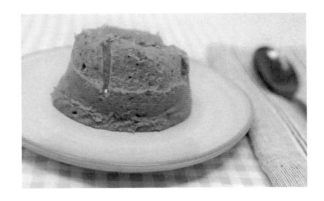

Ingredients

6 to 8 carrots, cut into 1-inch rounds (2 cups)
1 cup Bone Broth (page 19)

Instructions

Combine the carrots and broth in a pot over medium-high heat and boil for 15 minutes, until very soft.
Reserving roughly ½ cup of liquid, pour the carrots and broth into a food processor or blender.
Puree until smooth, adding some of the reserved broth until the puree reaches your desired creaminess.

You can't grow forward if you can't be honest about your faults.

CARAMELIZED ASPARAGUS

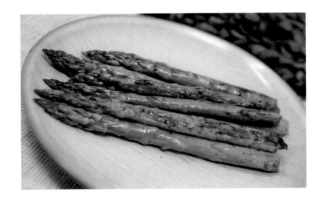

Ingredients

4 to 8 asparagus stalks
Pinch pink Himalayan sea salt
¼ teaspoon manuka honey, or maple syrup
1 teaspoon olive oil

Eat to aid your body. Not deprive it.

Instructions

In a bowl, toss the asparagus, salt, and honey together.
In a sauté pan on medium heat, heat the oil.
Add the asparagus and cook for 1 to 2 minutes, until caramelized.
*Try not to cook it any longer because the longer you cook asparagus, the more it loses its nutrients.

> *The more food is cooked, the more beneficial enzymes are cooked away with it. "Flash frying" asparagus will allow the nutrients to "activate" without cooking off their healthy enzymes.*

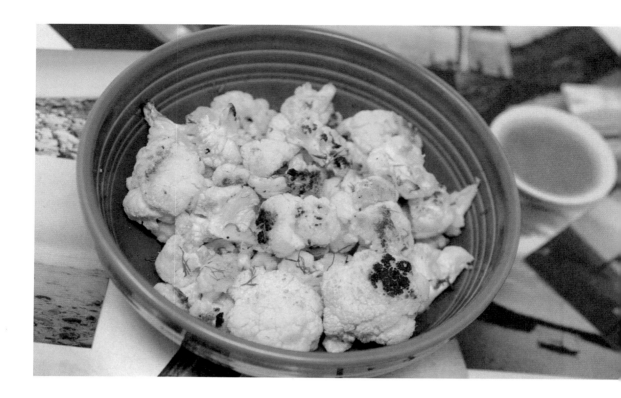

OVEN-FIRED CAULIFLOWER W/DILL

How hard are you willing to work? How much are you willing to sacrifice? To let go?

Ingredients

2 tablespoons olive oil

Juice of 1 medium lemon

1 tablespoon chopped fresh dill

1 teaspoon pink Himalayan sea salt

1 teaspoon ground turmeric

1 teaspoon ground ginger

1 medium cauliflower, cut into florets

Avoid getting stuck in routines (like a sweet potato every day). Too much of anything... never a good thing.

Instructions

Preheat the oven to 400°.

In a medium bowl, whisk together the oil, lemon juice, dill, salt, turmeric, and ginger.

Add the cauliflower and toss.

Spread out onto a baking sheet and bake for 20 minutes, mixing 2 or 3 times.

Remove and let cool for 2 to 3 minutes before serving.

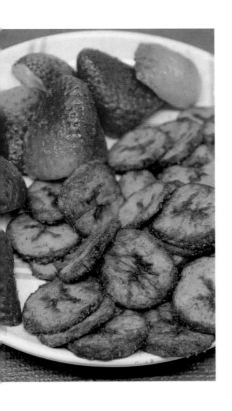

SWEET PLANTAINS

Ingredients

1 medium ripe plantain (dark yellow and blackening is best)
1 tablespoon coconut sugar
2 teaspoons ground cinnamon
2 teaspoons ground ginger
1 cup coconut oil

Instructions

Cut off the ends of the plantain and peel the outer shell off, just as you would a banana.
Use a mandolin or knife to slice the plantain into thin "chips."
Heat a sauté pan on medium-high heat and pour in enough coconut oil to cover the chips.
Add the plantain slices to the oil a few at a time to prevent them sticking together.
Fry until lightly golden brown, roughly 5 minutes.
Scoop the cooked chips onto a paper towel–lined plate and immediately toss with the sugar, cinnamon, and ginger.
Strain the oil into a glass jar and save.

CANDIED GINGER

Ingredients

¼ cup (2 ounces) sliced rounds fresh ginger
½ cup purified water
1 tablespoon manuka honey or maple syrup

Instructions

In a medium nonreactive pot over medium-high heat, combine the ginger, water, and honey and bring to a boil.
Reduce the heat to low and simmer for 10 minutes, stirring occasionally.
Scoop out the ginger pieces.
Strain the liquid into a glass jar and save to be used as **Ginger Simple Syrup** for mocktails and breakfast bowls.

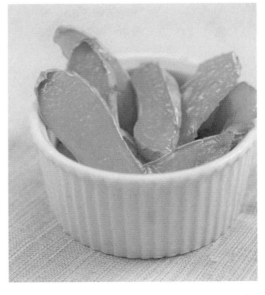

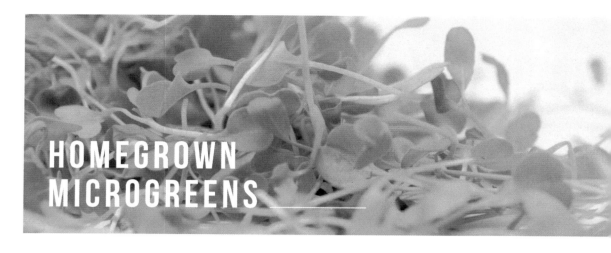

HOMEGROWN MICROGREENS

Ingredients

Organic seeds

Glass baking dish (or anything that is not plastic and at least 2 to 3 inches high and will fit on a windowsill or under a light), sanitized.

Organic soil (no synthetic fertilizers or water-retaining crystals and contains organic fertilizer such as compost or worm castings)

Paper towel (to cover while seeds are sprouting, or another tray, newspaper, or napkins)

Purified water

Watering can

Window or grow light

Trust yourself. Trust in time's healing. Demand trust from your food supply.

Instructions

Soak the seeds for a few hours or overnight.

Moisten the seedling mix until it can easily crumble but is not soggy or swampy.

Fill the container with 1 to 1½ inches of soil. Don't pack the soil. Keep it loose.

Level the soil with your hand or piece of cardboard.

Sprinkle the seeds evenly across the surface, so they are touching but not overlapping. This doesn't need to be perfect. Avoid packing them into the soil.

Cover the seeds with a moist paper towel and place in a warm, dark cupboard.

If everything remains moist, you don't need to do anything for 4 days. Spray the paper towel if you think more moisture is needed.

After the seeds have started to germinate, remove the cover and move the container into the light.

Continue to keep the growing sprouts moist. Water the soil from a watering can spout rather than spraying or misting the leaves. Watering the soil directly avoids growing mold instead of microgreens.

Start from the highest quality, whole, minimal ingredient foods and build from there.

RAW ST. TACOS

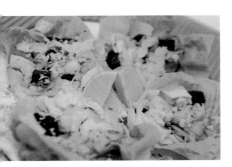

Ingredients

Riced broccoli

Minced leeks

Minced multicolored carrots

Diced peeled cucumber, seeds removed

Thinly sliced scallion (green part only)

1 teaspoon minced peeled fresh ginger

Butterhead lettuce cups

Diced roasted beets (page 14)

¼ to ½ medium avocado

Broccoli sprouts

Ground turmeric

Drizzle coconut aminos

Lime wedges

Optional

Fermented sauerkraut (note: avoid fermented foods until expansion phase)

Ground turkey (don't make it a habit!)

Instructions

Combine the broccoli rice, leeks, carrots, sauerkraut, cucumber, scallion, and ginger and layer in lettuce cups.

Top with beets, avocado, sprouts, and turmeric, drizzle with coconut aminos, and squeeze lime juice on top.

COCONUT FRIED RICE

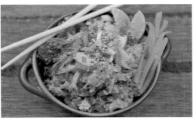

Ingredients

2 teaspoons olive oil

½ cup small broccoli florets

½ cup diced carrots

½ cup diced celery

¼ cup thinly sliced leeks

2 teaspoons minced peeled fresh ginger

2 cups riced cauliflower

2 tablespoons coconut aminos

Juice of ½ lime

2 teaspoons ground turmeric

½ cup arugula

8 to 14 fresh mint leaves

Toppings

Pinch microgreens

⅓ medium avocado

¼ cup chopped scallions

2 tablespoons sauerkraut

Coconut aminos (if needed)

1 tablespoon shelled hemp seeds

Instructions

Heat the oil in a large pan on medium heat.

Sauté the broccoli, carrots, celery, leeks, and ginger (and shrimp, if using) for 2 to 3 minutes or until slightly brown.

Mix in the cauliflower, coconut aminos, lime juice, and turmeric and sauté for 2 to 3 more minutes.

Add the arugula and mint. Cook, periodically stirring, for 3 to 5 more minutes or until the cauliflower is cooked to your liking. Scoop into a bowl and add your desired toppings.

Note: Hemp seeds are approved in small quantities. They are a rare seed that does not contain any phytic acid. They are high in protein and other essential nutrients, such as magnesium. Add when desired but avoid overindulgence.

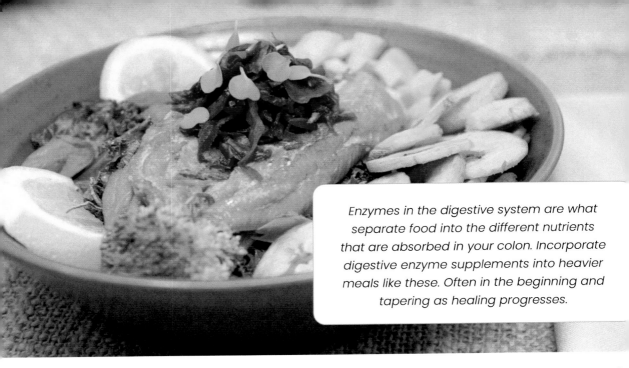

Enzymes in the digestive system are what separate food into the different nutrients that are absorbed in your colon. Incorporate digestive enzyme supplements into heavier meals like these. Often in the beginning and tapering as healing progresses.

KIPPER BOWL

If courage was easy and excuses were hard, accomplishments woul mean nothing.

Ingredients

½ tablespoon olive oil
½ cup broccoli florets
½ cup chopped kale
8 to 10 watercress leaves, minced
¼ cup microgreens
1 can kipper fillets (or sardines), strained
1/3 medium avocado
¼ cup sauerkraut
1 tablespoon coconut aminos
1 teaspoon ground turmeric
3 to 4 fresh sage leaves, minced
¼ lemon
Savory Plantain Chips (page 33)

Instructions

In a small sauté pan on medium heat, warm the olive oil.
Add the broccoli and kale, cover the pan, and sauté for 3 to 5 minutes, until the kale starts to wilt.
Transfer the broccoli and kale to a bowl and top with the watercress, microgreens, kippers, avocado, and sauerkraut.
Add the coconut aminos, turmeric, and sage.
Squeeze the lemon juice on top.
Line the rim of the bowl with plantain chips.

SOOTHING NOODLE PASTA

Ingredients

2 tablespoons olive oil

½ cup broccoli florets (fresh or thawed)

¼ cup thinly sliced leeks

4 to 6 asparagus stalks, woody ends snapped off, stalks halved

½ tablespoon minced fresh sage

1 medium spaghetti squash, roasted (page 14)

½ tablespoon coconut aminos

1 teaspoon lemon juice

Toppings

Thinly sliced scallion

¼ medium avocado, diced

1 tablespoon minced fresh basil

Pinch microgreens

Instructions

In a small pan on medium heat, warm the olive oil.

Add the broccoli, leeks, asparagus, and sage and partially cover the pan with a lid (leaving a slight opening for steam to escape).

Steam cook for 2 to 5 minutes or until tender, stirring every so often.

With a fork, scrape the squash into a bowl, forming "noodles."

Add the veggies, coconut aminos, and lemon juice and stir to evenly mix.

Separate servings into smaller bowls and add the toppings.

Not everything works out. That doesn't mean stop trying. Never stop trying.

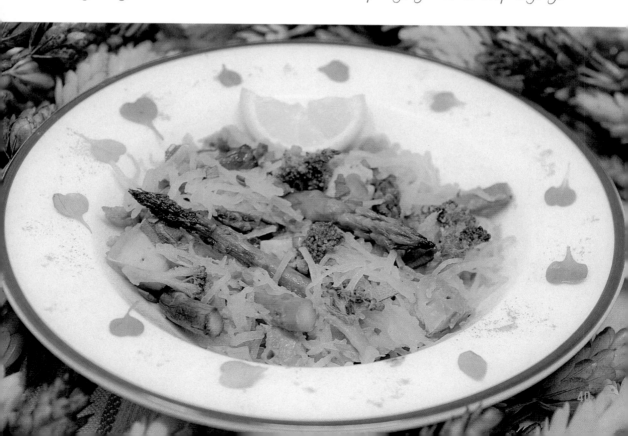

SKILLET STEAK

Ingredients

4 to 8 ounces top round steak, thinly sliced

Mmmm Marinade

4 to 6 Brussels sprouts

¼ acorn squash

Coconut oil, melted

1 tablespoon olive oil

Guacamole (page 33)

1 scoop sauerkraut

Broccoli sprouts

Instructions

Put the steak in a glass mason jar and combine with the marinade. Shake. Marinate in the refrigerator for at least 6 hours and up to 24 hours.

Preheat the oven to 375°. Line a baking sheet with tin foil.

Halve the acorn squash and baste with coconut oil.

Place the squash, cut-sides down, on the baking sheet and bake for 30 to 45 minutes or until easily pierced with a fork.

After 15 minutes of cooking time, prepare the Brussels sprouts (page 14) and add to the baking sheet in the oven. Cook for 15 to 30 minutes or until they reach your desired crispiness.

In a cast-iron skillet on medium heat, warm the olive oil.

Add the steak and marinade and cook until done to your liking.

Plate all the ingredients and serve with guacamole, sauerkraut, and sprouts.

STEAK SALAD

Ingredients

½ lemon

2 cups roughly chopped lacinato kale

4 ounces marinated steak

Guacamole (page 34)

¼ cup diced peeled

cucumber, seeds removed

1 medium beet, roasted and diced (page 14)

Pinch broccoli sprouts

½ cup Savory Plantain Chips (page 33)

Instructions

In a bowl, squeeze the lemon over the kale. Mix to evenly coat and refrigerate for 20 minutes.

Remove the kale from the refrigerator and top with the steak, guacamole, cucumber, beet, and sprouts.

Enjoy with a side of plantain chips.

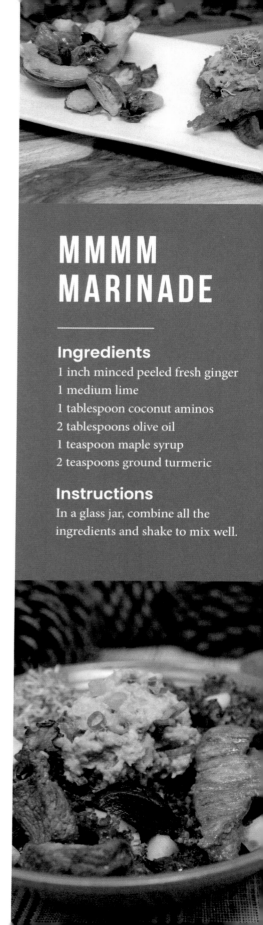

MMMM MARINADE

Ingredients

1 inch minced peeled fresh ginger

1 medium lime

1 tablespoon coconut aminos

2 tablespoons olive oil

1 teaspoon maple syrup

2 teaspoons ground turmeric

Instructions

In a glass jar, combine all the ingredients and shake to mix well.

HAPPY BUDDHA PASTA

Ingredients

- tablespoon olive oil
- cup diced carrots
- medium golden beets, roasted, peeled, and diced (page 14)
- tablespoon apple cider vinegar
- cup Bone Broth (page 19) or purified water
- teaspoons dried oregano
- teaspoon pink Himalayan sea salt
- or 5 leaves minced fresh sage
- tablespoon manuka honey
- medium spaghetti squash (or 2 cups cauliflower rice), roasted (page 14)
- Caramelized Asparagus (page 34)
- avocado, sliced
- minced basil, for garnish

Instructions

- a saucepan on medium heat, combine the oil and carrots.
- cook down until golden brown.
- combine the beets, carrots, apple cider vinegar, bone broth, oregano, salt, sage, and honey in a blender or processor and blend until smooth.
- with a fork, scrape the squash flesh into a bowl.
- should look like angel hair pasta.
- p with the sauce, asparagus, avocado, and basil.

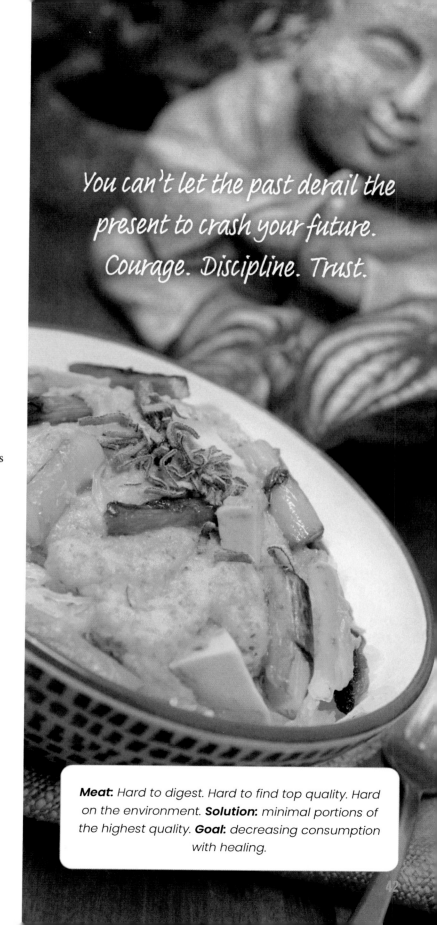

You can't let the past derail the present to crash your future. Courage. Discipline. Trust.

Meat: Hard to digest. Hard to find top quality. Hard on the environment. **Solution:** minimal portions of the highest quality. **Goal:** decreasing consumption with healing.

BUTTERNUT SALAD SAUTÉ

Ingredients
1 tablespoon olive oil
4 to 6 fresh asparagus stalks, tough ends snapped off
1 cup chopped kale
1 cup cubed roasted butternut squash (page 14)
1 tablespoon coconut aminos
8 to 10 watercress leaves, chopped
1 inch peeled cucumber, cubed and seeds removed
Pinch microgreens
¼ avocado, sliced

Dressing
1 tablespoon olive oil
Juice of ½ lemon
1 tablespoon manuka honey

Optional
1 can, or 6 ounces, salmon

Instructions
In a medium sauté pan on medium heat, heat the oil. Add the asparagus and kale, and flash-fry for 2 minutes (the longer you cook, the less nutrition and enzymes left to consume).
In a small glass jar, combine the dressing ingredients and shake until evenly mixed.
Transfer the squash, kale, and asparagus to a bowl. If using salmon, gently mix it in while drizzling on the coconut aminos.
Plate the mixture and top with the watercress, cucumber, microgreens, and avocado.

LIVER & LEEKS

Ingredients
4 to 8 ounces beef liver
1 cup coconut milk
1 tablespoon olive oil
1 cup thinly sliced leeks
2 teaspoons dried sage
½ tablespoon coconut aminos
1 medium butternut squash, roasted (page 14)
½ cup arugula
½ cup sauerkraut
1/3 medium avocado, sliced
¼ cup broccoli sprouts
¼ lemon

Optional
Sprouted brown rice or
1 scoop CauliMash (page 65)
(Note: these additions would no longer classify this recipe to this category.)

Instructions
In a glass storage container, combine the liver and coconut milk. Cover, shake, and refrigerate for at least 6 hours and up to overnight.
In a sauté pan on medium heat, warm the oil. Add the liver (not the liquid from the container), leeks, sage, and coconut aminos. Cook liver for 3 to 5 minutes, flip, and cook another 2 to 4 minutes or until cooked to your liking.
Plate the squash, arugula, liver, and leeks.
Top with the sauerkraut, avocado, and sprouts.
Squeeze the lemon over it all.

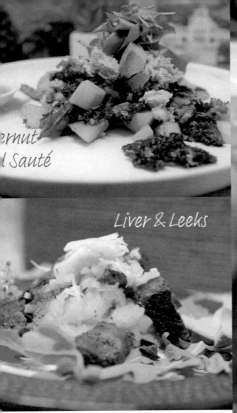

Liver & Leeks

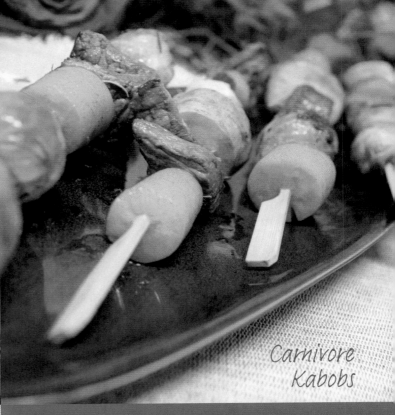

Carnivore
Kabobs

ARNIVORE
ABOBS

gredients
o 8 ounces sliced or cubed marinated
o round steak (page 41)
ussels sprouts, trimmed
medium sweet potato
carrot
rocado oil
esh rosemary
trus Ginger Glaze

ptional
Note: this addition reclassifies the
cipe as expansion phase)
rtobello mushroom, cubed

CITRUS GINGER GLAZE

Ingredients
½ tablespoon apple
cider vinegar
Juice and zest 1 lime
1 tablespoon minced
peeled fresh ginger
Juice of ½ medium orange
1 tablespoon olive oil

Instructions
In a small glass jar, combine
all the ingredients and shake
what your mama gave you
(or for at least 30 seconds).

Instructions
Turn the grill to medium heat.

Chop all the ingredients to roughly the same size.

Thread the steak, Brussels sprouts, sweet potato, and carrot
onto kabob sticks, alternating the order.

Baste with oil and sprinkle with rosemary.

Grill for 8 to 12 minutes, rotating the kabobs every so often.

When the sweet potato has softened, it's ready!

Plate with a side of citrus ginger glaze as a dipping sauce.

Deep breaths. Relax. You deserve it.

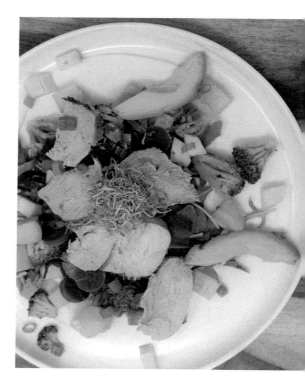

OVEN-ROASTED TURKEY BREAST

Ingredients
1 cup sliced carrots (1-inch rounds)
½ cup thinly sliced celery (2 stalks)
½ cup thinly sliced leeks (1 large leek)
½ cup Bone Broth (page 19)
1½ pounds bone-in turkey breast
3 tablespoons olive oil, divided
Juice of ¾ lemon, divided
1 medium butternut squash, halved lengthwise
½ cup steamed broccoli
1 cup arugula
3 to 5 pitted olives, sliced
¼ sliced avocado
1 inch peeled cucumber, diced and seeds removed
1 scallion, thinly sliced (green parts only)
Pinch broccoli sprouts

Optional
¼ cup kimchi (or sauerkraut variety)

Spices
Ground turmeric
Dried tarragon
Ground ginger
Dried sage

Meditation. Stretching. Yoga. Breathing. Walking.

Equally as important as food and supplements.

Instructions
Preheat the oven to 425°. Line a baking sheet with tin foil.

Line the bottom of a glass baking dish with the carrots, celery, leeks, and bone broth.

Peel back the turkey skin (keeping it attached on one side) and baste the flesh with 1 tablespoon of oil and two-thirds of the lemon juice. Then, rub on the spices and re-cover with the skin. Set it on the baking sheet.

Baste the cut sides of the squash with 1 tablespoon of olive oil and place cut-sides down on the baking sheet.

Cover the turkey and place it and the squash in the oven, immediately turning the heat down to 375°.

Bake for 45 minutes or until the internal temperature of the breast reaches 165° (checking from the center of the thickest part of the breast) and until the squash is easily pierced with a fork.

Steam the broccoli until soft, 4 to 5 minutes.

In a bowl, combine the arugula, olives, the remaining 1 tablespoon of olive oil, avocado, cucumber, remaining lemon juice, and scallion.

When the turkey is baked, remove and allow to rest for 10 to 15 minutes.

Halve the squash halves, plate one piece, and store the rest. Slice the turkey, divide into 4 portions, plate one, and store the rest.

Strain the remaining turkey liquid into a glass jar and use later for gravy with CauliMash (page 65). Save the turkey bone, freezing it for future use in Turkey Bone Broth (page 19).

Plate the salad, roasted veggies, and steamed broccoli.

Top with the sauerkraut and microgreens.

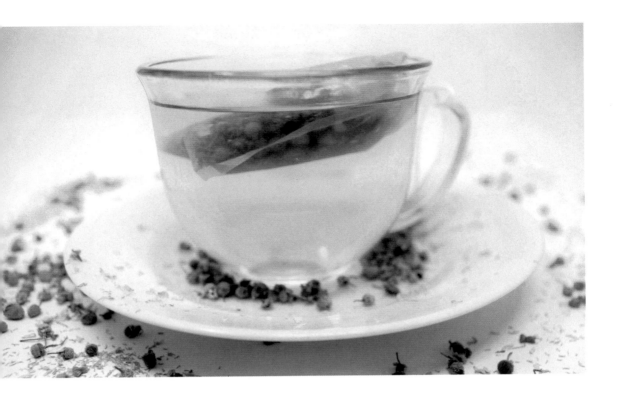

CHAMOMILE TEA

Did you meditate today? You're only lying to your progress. Nobody else.

Ingredients

Chamomile buds

Slice lemon

1 to 2 cups purified water

Instructions

Bring the water to a boil.

Place the chamomile buds in an unbleached tea bag and place in the water.

Squeeze in the lemon juice.

Let the bag steep for 4 to 6 minutes.

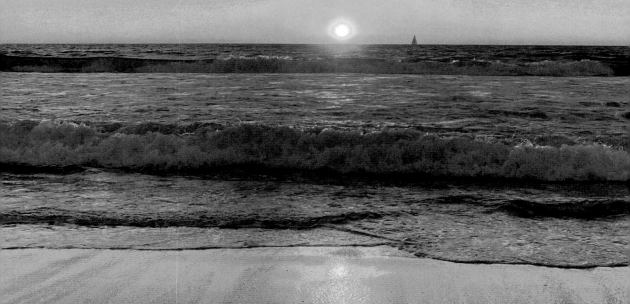

Walk the shore. Find your survivor's beauty.

THE EXPANSION PHASE

THE EXPANSION PHASE

These recipes are for when balance has been found, your body is calm, the supplement groundwork has taken hold, your foundation is established, and it's time to subtly expand. You're not yet ready to reintroduce the highest risk of trigger ingredients. But you are ready to widen nutritional variety and avoid complacency. Do not become dependent on these recipes. But be refreshed by their every-few-days delicious happiness offerings.

NOTES:
- *Exercise- Moderate exercise. 3-5 mile walks or 5,00-10,000 steps goal. This isn't strenuous. This is growth. Not exhaustion. Something outside. Hiking, biking, walking to the store, a walk with a loved one, or similar. After exercising, eat within 1 hour for the best results.*

- *Probiotics- Slowly start to reduce to 25-50 billion a day. Adjusting with your conditions comfort..*

This is forever a blessing.

Not a curse.

SUNRISE STIR-FRY

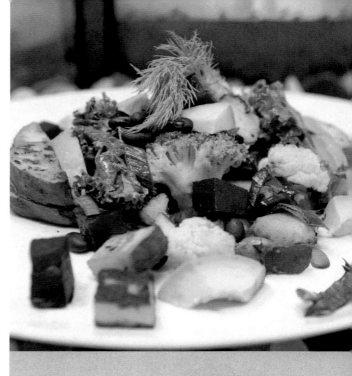

Ingredients

½ tablespoon coconut oil

1 medium mountain yam
(or ½ cup cubed squash), diced

Juice of ½ lime

½ teaspoon minced fresh dill

1 teaspoon ground ginger

1 teaspoon ground turmeric

1/3 cup broccoli florets

1/3 cup cauliflower florets

¼ cup sliced leeks

½ cup chopped kale

¼ cup diced roasted beets (page 14)

2 tablespoons cooked black beans (page 56)

1/3 avocado, sliced

Chopped scallion (green parts only)

Pinch sprouts

Sweet Ginger Sauce (page 49)

SWEET GINGER SAUCE

Ingredients

2 tablespoons coconut aminos

½ tablespoon ground ginger

1 teaspoon lime juice

1 teaspoon ground turmeric

Instructions

In a small bowl, combine all the ingredients and stir until evenly blended.

Instructions

In a cast-iron skillet on medium heat, warm the coconut oil.

Add the yam to the pan with the lime juice, dill, ginger, and turmeric.

Toss until evenly coated and cover with a lid for 3 to 5 minutes.

Add the broccoli, cauliflower, and leeks. Cover and sauté for 3 to 5 minutes, adding more oil if needed.

Add the kale, cover, and saute for 3 to 5 more minutes, adding more oil if needed.

Transfer the stir-fry to a plate and top with the beets, beans, avocado, scallion, sprouts, and sweet ginger sauce.

There are over 30 strains of beneficial probiotic bacteria and not all are friendly to your specific conditions. Choose wisely.

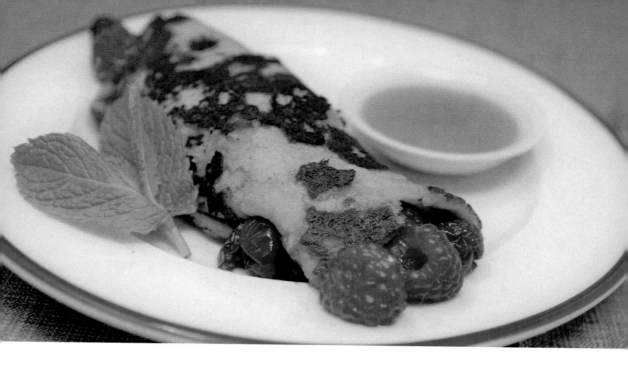

CREPE ROLL-UPS

Ingredients

½ cup cooked peeled sweet potato (or squash)

1 medium ripe banana

1/3 cup coconut flour
(or more for right consistency)

1 cup purified water

1 scoop (20 g) collagen peptide powder

1½ tablespoons apple cider vinegar

½ tablespoon maple syrup, or manuka honey

1 teaspoon ground cinnamon

½ tablespoon coconut oil, or avocado oil

1 tablespoon Cranberry Sauce (page 45)

½ cup raspberries

Optional

Exchange the cranberries and raspberries for blueberries or pomegranate seeds.

Rotate the sweet potatoes, making sure you're not consuming too much in a day or too much of one kind. Variety builds balance.

Instructions

Preheat the oven to 375°. Wash the sweet potato and bake for 45 minutes.

Combine the banana, coconut flour, water, sweet potato, collagen peptide powder, apple cider vinegar, honey, and cinnamon in a blender or food processor. Blend until smooth.

Heat a pan on medium heat and coat with the oil.

Pour about 1/3 cup of batter into the pan.

Lift and tilt until the batter spreads as thin as possible.

Cook for 2 to 3 minutes until the edges release and you can slide in a spatula.

Flip and cook for another 2 minutes.

Remove and repeat with the remaining batter.

Fill with the cranberry sauce and raspberries, and roll.

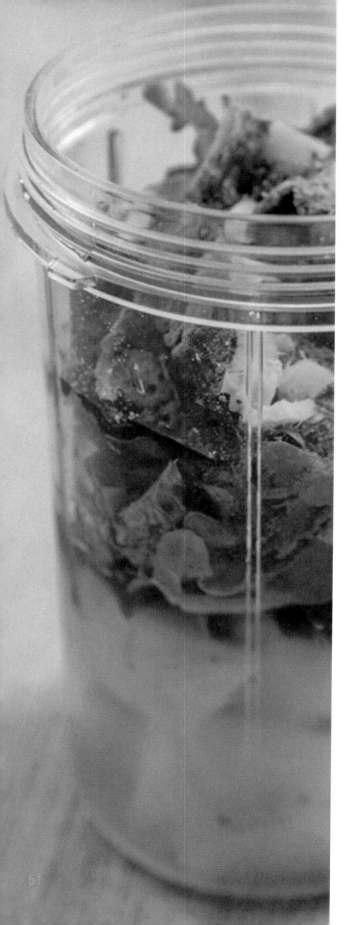

GREEN PINEAPPLE SMOOTHIE

Ingredients

½ cup frozen pineapple chunks
½ teaspoon ground turmeric
½ teaspoon minced fresh peeled ginger
½ teaspoon ground cinnamon
½ cup pressed kale
½ cup cold purified water
Pinch pink Himalayan sea salt
2 or 3 ices cubes purified water

Optional

1 scoop (20 g) collagen peptide powder

Instructions

Combine all the ingredients in a
smoothie maker or blender.
Blend until creamy smooth.

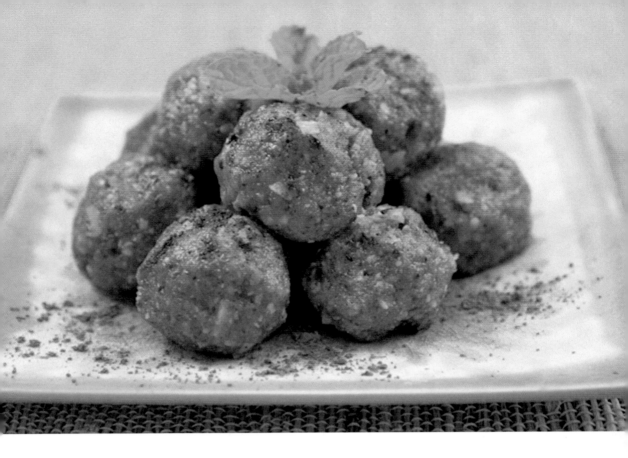

PUMPKIN PROTEIN BALLS

Ingredients

½ cup pumpkin puree

2 scoops (40g or 3 tablespoons) collagen peptide powder

4 tablespoons coconut flour

1 teaspoon ground cinnamon

2 medjool dates

2 tablespoons pomegranate seeds

1 tablespoon minced peeled fresh ginger

Pack a piece of fruit, 2 to 4 protein balls, and a bottle of purified water and enjoy after a low-impact hike somewhere new.

Instructions

Combine the pumpkin puree, collagen peptide powder, coconut flour, cinnamon, and dates in a processer and pulse until thoroughly mixed.

Transfer to a bowl and fold in the pomegranate seeds and ginger until evenly mixed.

With a spoon, scoop and roll into 1-inch balls.

Place in the refrigerator for 1 hour before serving.

Note:

A serving of 1 to 3 at a time max. Combine with a piece of fruit or as another component. Not a meal. That's the overindulgence.

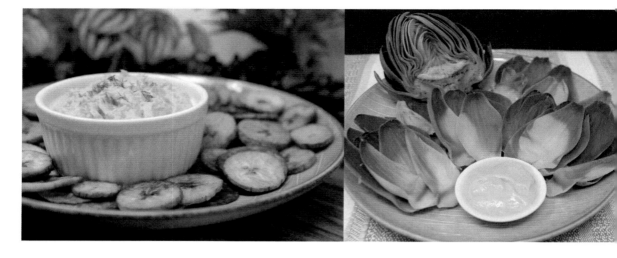

CITRUS ARTICHOKE HUMMUS

Ingredients

1 cup globe artichoke hearts
1 garlic clove
½ avocado, sliced
1 tablespoon olive oil
1 tablespoon lemon juice
1 tablespoon minced fresh dill
1 serving Savory Plantain Chips (page 33)

Instructions

Rinse, strain, and carefully press and blot the artichoke hearts to remove all excess liquid (so the hummus isn't watery).
Combine the artichoke and garlic into a food processor, and pulse until roughly chopped.
Add the oil and lemon juice, and blend until creamy.
Stir in the dill and serve with your favorite side.

ARTICHOKE DIPPERS

Ingredients

1 fresh artichoke
Purified water
1 teaspoon pink Himalayan sea salt
1 recipe Lemon-Garlic Aioli
½ lemon

Instructions

Cut the tips of the artichoke leaves and stem. If large, cut in half for faster cooking.
In a large pot over high heat, bring water to a boil.
Add the salt and artichoke, and boil for 30 to 45 minutes or until easily pierced with a fork.
Squeeze on lemon juice and serve with the aioli.

LEMON-GARLIC AIOLI

Ingredients

½ cup Avocado Mayo (page 25)
1 tablespoon lemon juice
2 garlic cloves, minced

Instructions

In a small bowl or processor mix all the ingredients together thoroughly.

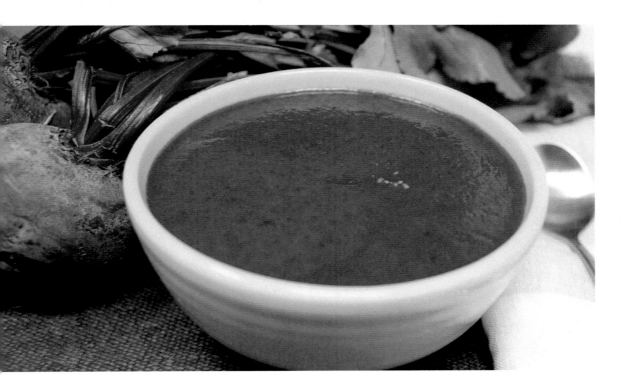

BACK TO YOUR BEETROOTS SOUP

"Landmines": the situations of vulnerability that justify progress-killing choices. More self-respect, more self-success."

ngredients

medium beets

tablespoons olive oil

½ cup thinly sliced leeks

garlic cloves, minced (if still following FODMAP restrictions, omit)

cup cranberries

cups Bone Broth (page 19)

tablespoon lemon juice

tablespoon fresh minced dill, plus 1 teaspoon for garnish

tablespoon minced peeled fresh ginger

teaspoon ground turmeric

Pinch pink Himalayan sea salt

Instructions

Peel and dice the beets.

In a large pot over medium heat, warm the olive oil.

Add the leeks and garlic and sauté until soft, 3 to 5 minutes.

Add the beets and cranberries and sauté for another 4 minutes.

Add the broth, stir, and cover the pot.

Lightly simmer until the beets are tender, about 40 minutes.

Let cool for 20 to 30 minutes.

Transfer to a processor or blender. Add the lemon juice, 1 tablespoon of dill, ginger, turmeric, and salt and puree until it reaches your desired creaminess.

Garnish with the remaining 1 teaspoon of dill.

Identify, prepare and eliminate landmine scenarios.

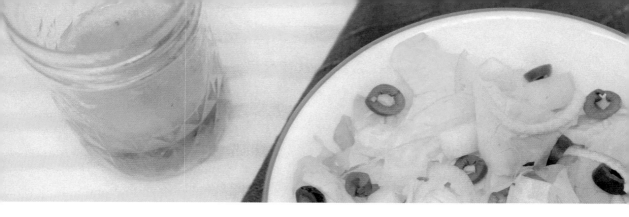

GREEK SALAD

Ingredients

2 tablespoons unpitted Kalamata olives
½ head butterhead lettuce, roughly chopped
3 tablespoons thinly sliced red onion
¼ medium peeled cucumber, diced and
seeds removed
Greek Dressing

Note: If following strict FODMAP
restrictions, replace the onion with leek.
Green parts only.

Instructions

Remove the pits from the olives and slice.
In a large bowl, toss together the olives,
lettuce, onion, and cucumber.
Slowly drizzle with dressing and continue to
toss until coated.

GREEK DRESSING

Ingredients

¼ cup olive oil
Juice of ½ medium lemon
1 tablespoon apple cider vinegar
1 garlic clove, minced (if following
strict FODMAP protocol, omit)
Pinch pink Himalayan sea salt
½ teaspoon dried oregano
3 Kalamata olives, minced

Instructions

In a glass jar, combine all the
ingredients and shake, shake, shake
for 30 seconds to 1 minute.

GARLIC VINAIGRETTE

Ingredients

½ cup olive oil
1 tablespoon apple cider vinegar
Juice of ½ lemon
½ teaspoon pink Himalayan sea salt
1½ teaspoons manuka honey (or maple syrup)
1 garlic clove, minced
1 teaspoon black pepper
1 teaspoon ground turmeric

Instructions

Combine all the ingredients in a glass
jar and shake until evenly mixed.

Perception toward action heals or steals nutrition.

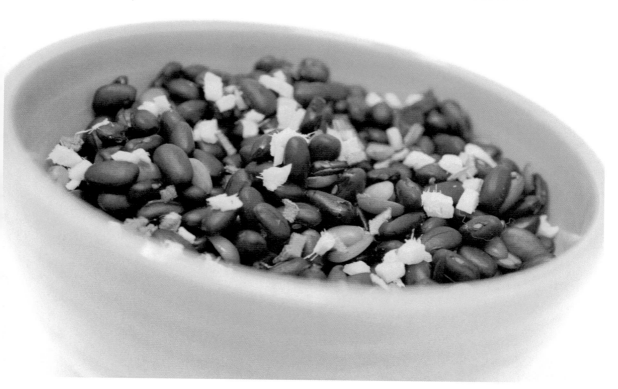

DEACTIVATED BEANS

Ingredients

1 cup black beans

2 cups purified water

1 tablespoon apple cider vinegar

1 cup Bone Broth (page 19)

1 to 2 teaspoons pink Himalayan sea salt

2 teaspoons minced fresh sage

1 to 2 teaspoons minced peeled fresh ginger

2 teaspoons ground turmeric

Optional

Tired of black beans?

Try kidney or pinto.

Instructions

Soak the beans in 1 cup of purified water and the apple cider vinegar for at least 8 hours and up to overnight. Thoroughly rinse the beans and combine with the remaining 1 cup of water, broth, and salt in a pot over high heat. Cover and bring to a boil.

Reduce to a simmer and uncover.

Cook for 1½ to 2 hours until the beans are tender.

If at any time your beans go dry, add more broth to slightly cover the beans.

Strain and season with the sage, ginger, and turmeric.

Avoid garbanzo beans. They cause disruptions in the gastrointestinal tract of people with intestinal issues and trigger system flushing.

Sprouted foods contain dense amounts of vital nutrients and enhanced bioavailability.

Create love, give love, be loved.

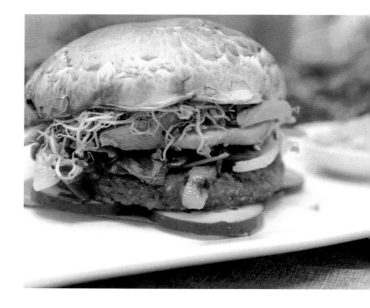

SPROUTED BLACK BEAN BURGER

Ingredients

1 cup Deactivated Beans (page 56)
¼ cup cooked brown rice
2 tablespoons olive oil, plus more for coating pan
1 tablespoon apple cider vinegar
2 teaspoons coconut aminos
1 teaspoon manuka honey (or maple syrup)
2 teaspoons dried oregano
1 teaspoon ground turmeric
1 teaspoon ground ginger
1 teaspoon pink Himalayan sea salt
2 to 3 tablespoons sprouted almond flour
2 tablespoons minced carrots
2 tablespoons minced yellow onion
2 tablespoons minced celery
1 garlic clove, minced

Toppings

½ collard green leaf
Portobello Mushroom Bun
Sliced avocado
Grilled onion
Broccoli sprouts
Sliced peeled cucumber, seeds removed
Beet sauerkraut
Watercress

NOTE: Get creative with toppings. But stay within the boundaries!!

Instructions

In a bowl, combine the black beans and rice, and mash together.

Add 2 tablespoons of olive oil, apple cider vinegar, coconut aminos, honey, oregano, turmeric, ginger, salt, and almond flour, and mix together.

Once mixed, gently stir in the carrots, celery, onion, and garlic.

In a large saute pan on medium heat, warm the oil.

Form the mixture to your desired patty shape and add it to the pan.

Cover and fry until the bottom turns light brown. Flip, cover, and cook for 3 to 5 more minutes. Be careful not to overcook and burn the patty.

On a plate, fold the collard green leaf to your desired shape and stack with the patty and your desired ingredients. End with portobello bun or a replacement that works for your current condition.

PORTOBELLO MUSHROOM BUN

Ingredients
tablespoons olive oil
or 2 large portobello mushrooms

Instructions
reheat the oven to 400°. Line a baking sheet
ith parchment paper and evenly drizzle
ith oil to coat.
ash the mushrooms in cold water and dry.
venly coat the bottom side of the
ushrooms with oil and place top-side down.
ake for 8 to 10 minutes. Flip and bake for
other 8 to 10 minutes, until fork tender.

*Risky ingredients: *Nightshades for high antinutrient content *Mushrooms because of fungus and mold exposure *Garlic and onions are high–FODMAP foods (page 11)*

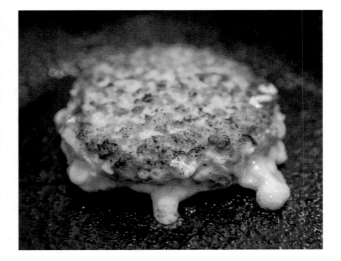

SALMON CAKES

Ingredients
1 (6-ounce) can salmon
¼ cup pumpkin puree
1 tablespoon coconut flour
½ teaspoon lemon juice
Pinch pink Himalayan sea salt
Pinch ground turmeric
½ tablespoon minced fresh sage
1 scallion, chopped
½ tablespoon minced fresh dill or 2 teaspoons dried
1 tablespoon melted coconut oil
Lemon wedges for serving
¼ cup Lemon-Garlic Aioli (page 53)

Instructions
Preheat the oven to 400°.
Drain the salmon and remove any bones. Place it in a large bowl and mix with the pumpkin puree, coconut flour, lemon juice, salt, turmeric, sage, scallion, and dill. Evenly coat a cast-iron skillet with the coconut oil and turn the heat to medium.
With a ¼-cup measuring cup, scoop out some salmon and mold it to your desired burger shape.
Fry for 5 minutes, then flip the cake with a spatula and fry for another 5 to 10 minutes or until golden brown. Serve with a lemon wedge and the aioli.

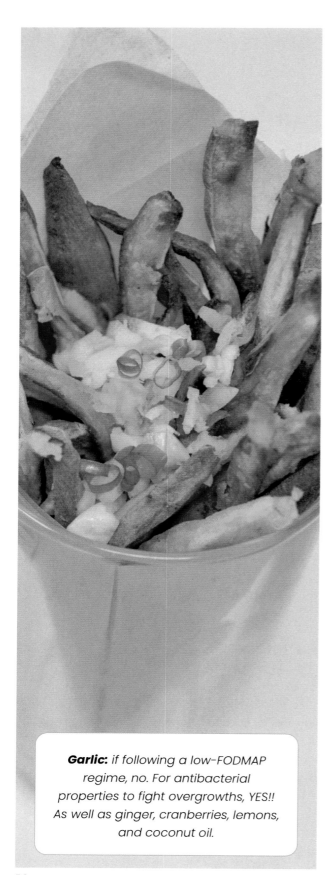

GARLIC FRIES

Ingredients

1 medium sweet potato
Avocado oil
2 teaspoons fresh minced garlic

Optional

Sweet Ginger Sauce (page 49)

Instructions

Preheat the oven to 400°. Line a baking sheet
with parchment paper.
Slice the sweet potatoes into long strips.
In a bowl, toss the sweet potatoes and some
avocado oil until fully coated.
Evenly spread on the baking sheet.
Bake for 20 to 30 minutes or until the sweet
potatoes turn golden brown.
Bowl and top with the garlic, scallion, and
salt. Serve with sweet ginger sauce, if desired.

Garlic: if following a low–FODMAP
regime, no. For antibacterial
properties to fight overgrowths, YES!!
As well as ginger, cranberries, lemons,
and coconut oil.

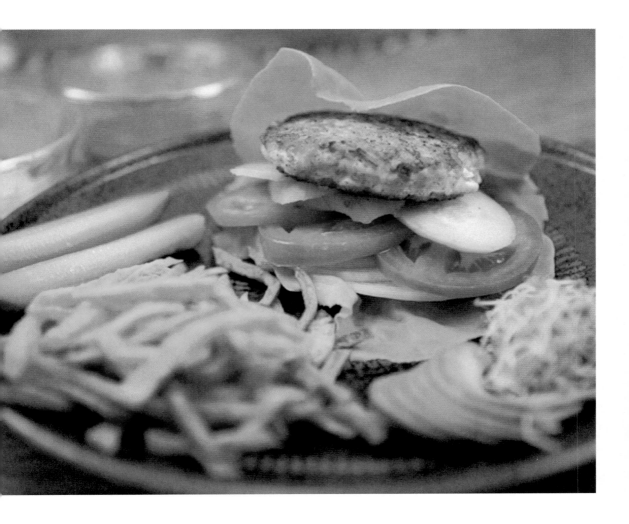

SEA BURGERS

Toppings
Butterhead lettuce leaves
Sliced cucumber
Sliced avocado
Broccoli sprouts
Lemon-Garlic Aioli (page 53)

If you see it as daunting, it'll always be daunting.

If you see it as exciting, it'll be exciting.

Optional
Onion (only if high-FODMAP foods can be tolerated).
Sliced tomato (this nightshade addition would reclassify the recipe to Reintroduction and only in small amounts if allergy tests prove no allergen to your body).
Pickle spears

BEETGHETTI DINNER

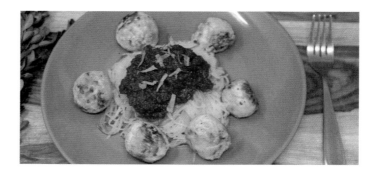

Ingredients

1 medium spaghetti squash, roasted, (page 14) or 2 cups cauliflower rice
3 medium beets, roasted (page 14)
1½ tablespoons olive oil, divided
¾ cup diced carrots
¼ cup thinly sliced leeks
2 garlic cloves, minced
½ tablespoon apple cider vinegar
2 tablespoons purified water
2 teaspoons dried oregano
½ teaspoon pink Himalayan sea salt
4 to 5 fresh sage leaves, minced
1 tablespoon manuka honey

Topping

Minced basil

Instructions

In a saucepan on medium heat, combine the olive oil, carrots, leeks, and garlic.
Cook until golden brown. Transfer to a blender or processor.
Add the apple cider vinegar, water, oregano, salt, sage, and honey and blend until smooth.
Return the sauce to the pan (scraping the sides of the blender) and heat on low for 10 to 15 minutes.
With a fork, scrape the spaghetti squash flesh into a bowl.
It should look like angel hair pasta at this point.
Top with the beets and sauce.

Note: If using cauliflower rice, simply combine the oil and rice in a saucepan on medium heat and cook until light brown.

Optional

Add Flatbread (page 84) and Pesto (page 84).

TURKEY MEATBALLS

Stay educated on the deceit. What's exposed today will be renamed tomorrow.

Ingredients

1 pound ground turkey breast
1 tablespoon dried oregano
½ tablespoon dried rosemary
2 garlic cloves, minced
Pinch pink himalayan sea salt
1 tablespoon coconut aminos
2 teaspoons ground turmeric
2 tablespoons olive oil

Instructions

In a bowl, combine the turkey, oregano, rosemary, garlic, salt, coconut aminos, and turmeric and mix thoroughly.
Heat the oil in a sauté pan on medium heat.
Form the mixture into meatballs and cook, rotating, until golden brown.
If combining this recipe with Beetghetti Dinner, this is the time where you combine the meatballs with the pasta sauce in the pan and let it cook on low heat for 10 to 15 minutes.

LIVER & ONIONS

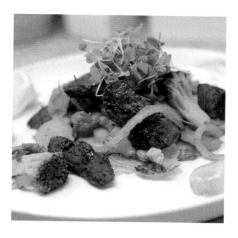

Ingredients

4 to 8 ounces beef liver

3 tablespoons olive oil, divided, plus more for drizzling garlic

1 tablespoon coconut aminos

Juice of ½ medium lemon

1 head garlic

3 to 6 Brussels sprouts, halved

¼ cup broccoli florets

¼ cup sliced carrot rounds

¼ medium sweet onion, sliced

1 teaspoon ground turmeric

1 teaspoon dried rosemary

Microgreens

Instructions

In a container, combine the liver, 1 tablespoon of olive oil, coconut aminos, and lemon juice.

Toss to evenly coat and place in the refrigerator for at least 6 hours and up to overnight.

Preheat the oven to 350°.

Cut the top off the garlic head and drizzle with a dab of olive oil. Wrap in tin foil and roast for 30 minutes.

Toss the Brussels sprouts, carrots, and broccoli, with 1 tablespoon of olive oil. Spread evenly on a baking sheet. Roast for 20 to 25 minutes or until browned.

In a sauté pan on medium heat, warm the remaining 1 tablespoon of olive oil.

Add the liver, onion, turmeric, and rosemary and cook for 5 to 8 minutes, stirring periodically.

Plate the veggies, liver and onions, and 2 to 4 cloves of roasted garlic.

Top with the microgreens.

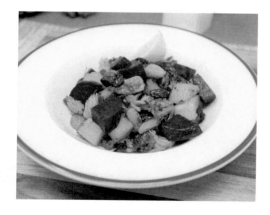

ROASTED VEGGIE BOWL

Ingredients

1 medium acorn squash

2 garlic cloves, minced

½ tablespoon coconut oil

1 cup halved, or shaven, Brussels sprouts

1 cup chopped broccoli florets

2 medium beets, chopped

2 teaspoons minced fresh sage

1 teaspoon ground turmeric

Instructions

Preheat the oven to 375°.

Line a baking sheet with tin foil.

Toss all the ingredients together in a small bowl then spread in a single layer on the baking sheet.

Bake until light brown and tender, mixing every so often, 15 to 20 minutes.

Bowl, or plate, and serve.

Optional

Pair this recipe with another side or two, or on CauliMash (page 65) or on top of a salad.

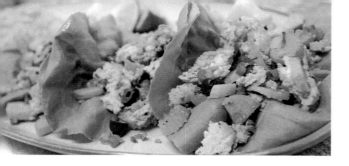

YUMMY TUMMY TACOS

Ingredients

1 cup cooked brown rice
1 cup purified water
1 tablespoon apple cider vinegar
1 cup Bone Broth (page 19) or 2 cups purified water
½ tablespoon olive oil, plus more to coat the pan
1 pound ground turkey
¼ cup diced sweet onion
1 medium carrot, diced
½ celery stalk, diced
1 inch minced peeled fresh ginger
1 teaspoon ground turmeric
½ tablespoon dried rosemary
1 teaspoon dried tarragon
1 tablespoon coconut aminos
Butterhead lettuce leaves

Toppings

Finely sliced scallion
Microgreens
Avocado, sliced
4 to 6 unpitted black olives, pitted by you and sliced
1 medium lime

Optional

Sauerkraut

Instructions

In a glass container, soak the rice in the water and apple cider vinegar for at least 6 hours and up to overnight.

Strain, wash, and place the rice with the bone broth in a small pot on medium heat. Cover the pot (leaving a small opening for steam to release).

When the water starts to boil, reduce the heat to low and simmer until all the water is absorbed and the rice is soft, roughly 20 minutes. Avoid stirring!

Coat a large saucepan on medium heat with the oil.

In a bowl, mix together the turkey, onion, carrot, celery, ginger, turmeric, rosemary, tarragon, and coconut aminos.

Transfer the mixture to the pan and flatten.

Prep the toppings while the meat cooks.

Set up your taco assembly line and enjoy with your loved ones.

BASE GROUND TURKEY

Ingredients

½ tablespoon olive oil
12 to 16 ounces fresh ground turkey breast (not packaged)
½ lime
1 tablespoon minced peeled fresh ginger
½ tablespoon ground turmeric
½ tablespoon dried tarragon
1 tablespoon coconut aminos

Optional

½ tablespoon dried sage
½ tablespoon dried oregano

Instructions

In a glass pan on medium heat, warm the oil.

In a bowl, combine the remaining ingredients and thoroughly mix with your hands.

Put the mixture in the pan and flatten it evenly.

Cook for 2 to 4 minutes.

Flip and cook until finished, breaking it up to your desired size with a spatula.

BAKE IN A BAG

The process is... a third mindset, a third movement, a third diet.

Ingredients

1 cup cooked brown rice

1 cup purified water

1 tablespoon apple cider vinegar, plus 2 teaspoons

1 scallion

4 or 5 asparagus stalks

½ cup small broccoli florets

3 to 5 artichoke hearts

1 large carrot

½ cup pressed kale or baby spinach

3 or 4 thinly sliced lemon ovals

1 tablespoon olive oil

2 fresh rosemary sprigs

1 teaspoon dried thyme

2 teaspoons dried dill

Nonstick unbleached parchment medium roasting bag

2 cups Bone Broth (page 19), or purified water

Optional

6 ounces salmon

½ tablespoon coconut aminos

Feeling sorry for yourself heals nothing. What you have is it. And. It. Is. Beautiful.

Instructions

In a glass container, soak the rice in the purified water and 1 tablespoon of apple cider vinegar for at least 6 hours and up to 24 hours.

Preheat the oven to 400°.

In a bowl, combine the scallion, asparagus, broccoli, artichoke hearts, and carrot and mix with the remaining 2 teaspoons of apple cider vinegar, olive oil, rosemary, thyme, and dill.

Line the bottom of the roasting bag with the kale.

Add the mixed ingredients.

Top with the lemon slices.

Bake for 30 minutes.

While the vegetables are roasting, drain and wash the rice.

In a small pot, combine the rice and bone broth. Bring to a boil then reduce the heat to a simmer.

Cover with the lid slightly angled to let steam out. Cook for 20 to 30 minutes, until the broth is absorbed.

Remove the roasting bag and carefully cut open with scissors.

Scoop the desired amount of rice into a bowl and top with veggies.

Strain the salmon from the can and place on top of the veggies.

Drizzle with the coconut aminos.

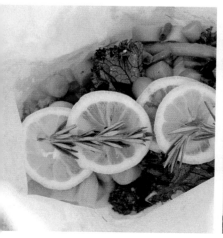

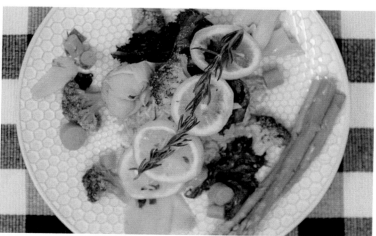

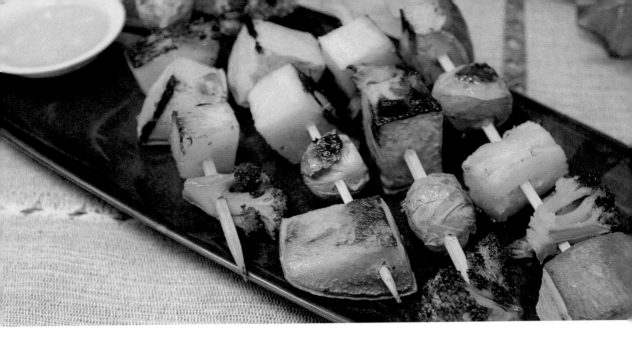

HERBIVORE KABOBS

Ingredients

1 medium sweet potato
Brussels sprouts
Cubed fresh pineapple
Portobello or shiitake mushrooms
Broccoli florets
Avocado oil
Citrus Ginger Glaze (page 44)

Instructions

Turn the grill to medium heat.
Chop the sweet potato, Brussels sprouts, pineapple, and mushrooms to roughly the same size and thread onto kabob sticks, alternating the order.
Baste with oil.
Grill for 8 to 12 minutes, rotating the kabobs every so often.
When the sweet potato has softened, it's ready!
Plate with a side of Citrus Ginger Glaze as a dipping sauce.

CAULIMASH

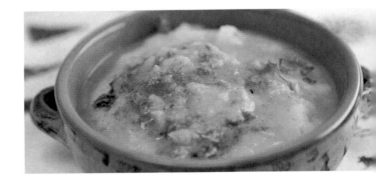

Ingredients

1 cup purified water
3 cups Bone Broth (page 19)
1 head cauliflower
Pinch pink Himalayan sea salt
1 tablespoon olive oil

Topping

Gravy
1 or 2 scallions, thinly sliced

Instructions

Combine the water and bone broth in a medium pot on high heat. Bring to a boil.
Add the cauliflower and reduce the heat to low.
Simmer until the cauliflower softens, 6 to 8 minutes.
Strain, reserving 1 cup of liquid for the blending process.
Combine the cauliflower, salt, and olive oil in a blender.
Blend until it reaches your desired creaminess, adding 1 tablespoon of reserved liquid at a time, if necessary.
Serve topped with gravy and the scallions.

AL'S BLUEBERRY PIE

Crust

1 cup plus 2 tablespoons coconut flour or
¾ cup white rice flour with ¼ cup plus 2
tablespoons coconut flour
½ cup olive oil
2 to 3 tablespoons purified water

Filling

1 tablespoon manuka honey or 1½
tablespoons organic maple syrup
1 tablespoon ground cinnamon
Juice and zest of 1 medium lemon
8 cups blueberries
½ tablespoon coconut flour

*If desiring a more personal pie size,
for portion control and to avoid
overconsumption, simply use a 6-inch
pie dish and cut the ingredients in
half. Prepare it the same way.*

Instructions

Crust

Preheat the oven to 375°.
Combine the crust ingredients in a bowl and hand
mix until it forms a dough-like consistency, adding
the water slowly as you go.
In an 8- or 9-inch pie plate, press the dough to
form an even crust.
Bake for 20 minutes, until light golden brown.
Transfer the pie plate to a wire rack to cool while
you make the filling.

Filling

Combine all the ingredients in a small saucepan
on medium-high heat and bring to a boil.
Immediately after reaching a boil, turn off the heat
and set the pan to the side.
Gently stir to combine.

Pie

Spread the filling over the crust and smooth.
Bake for 5 minutes, turn off the oven, and let the
pie cool inside the oven for 30 minutes or so.
Note: Take any excess blueberry juice and store as
Blueberry Simple Syrup for a later topping for
oatmeal, in a mocktail, or on top of The Classic
(page 23).

*You are the culmination of the five closest
people to you. Choose wisely. Value
immensely. Share their pie. :)*

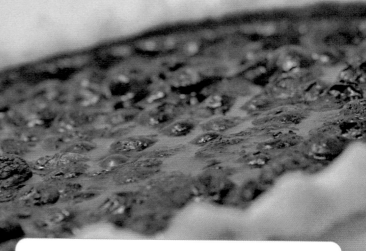

GRAVY

Ingredients

Baked turkey drippings (see page 44)
½ cup Bone Broth (page 19)
tablespoons coconut flour

Optional

¼ cup chopped mushrooms

Instructions

In a medium pan on medium heat, combine
the ingredients and bring to a gentle simmer.
Stir to thoroughly combine.
Season to your liking with any of the
approved spices (see page 7).
When the gravy thickens, it's ready.

*Traditional pumpkin pie: eggs, dairy, gluten,
antinutrients, preservatives, sugar, and endless
amounts of gut-irritating ingredients and
genetically engineered substances.*

STRAWBERRY-ORANGE

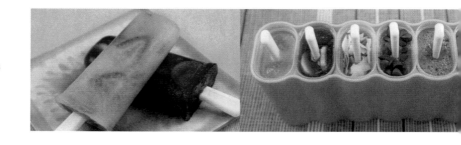

Ingredients

Fresh sliced strawberries
Sliced oranges
Purified water

Instructions

Into a glass, squeeze the oranges and mix in
purified water.
Creatively layer strawberries up the popsicle mold
and pour orange juice on top to the desired spot.
Position the sticks.
Freeze for at least an hour, until solid.
Note: Makes 3 to 4 popsicles

*Immune system—healing happy chemicals:
endorphins, dopamine, serotonin. Debilitating
stress chemical: cortisol. Everything else could
be perfect, but what fills your day dictates what
flows through the body and helps or exposes
the system.*

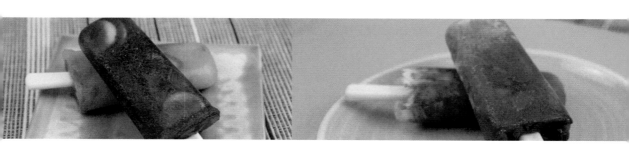

BANANA-POM

Ingredients

¼-inch-thick banana slices
Pomegranate juice

Instructions

Drop the banana slices one by one,
alternating directions, into the popsicle
mold and fill with pomegranate juice.
Position the sticks.
Freezer for at least an hour, until solid.

BLUEBERRY-GINGER

Ingredients

¼ cup ginger simple syrup
(see page 35)
½ cup blueberries
¼ avocado

*Life is where you
are right now.*

Instructions

After straining the simple syrup into a storage glass, let
cool and then combine in a blender with the blueberries
and avocado and blend until smooth.
Pour into popsicle molds.
Position the sticks.
Freeze for at least an hour, until solid.

THE REINTRODUCTION PHASE

"Avoid justification's trap of overindulging because of a first try success. You know this. So stop testing the boundaries and live in the beauty."

THE REINTRODUCTION PHASE

The book is yours. These recipes are dedicated for the times when order has been restored, expanded ingredients have been building strength, and your body is now healed enough to test out small amounts of other ingredients at a time. The strategy with these recipes is every once in a while, and not continuously repeating. These recipes contain an expanded menu of nutritious and staple ingredients, but the ingredients are possible disruptors if you still have lingering issues anywhere along the gastrointestinal tract. Ingredients of this nature are known as high FODMAP and fructose-dominant fruits and vegetables. Always c onsume in tolerable quantities for your conditions.

A majority of these recipes, if not treated properly, contain antinutrients that will cause disruptions and inflammatory damage along the digestive tract, blocking key nutrients from being absorbed. Antinutrients are mainly found in nuts, seeds, grains, and legumes. They are the shielding layer defending the seed so that it can achieve its one goal: germination. Unfortunately, our bodies no longer possess the enzymes for digesting them. Especially inflamed bodies. My strategy, when I feel comfortable in this phase, is to consume small amounts, spaced out, in rotation and for nutritional balance. The more consumed in a short period of time, the more strain and wearing. There is no wondering "if…" or "will it…?" with antinutrients, just damage. Healthy or not.

You've worked too hard to get here and give it up. So stay responsible and enjoy the right kind of treat with one of these delicious recipes.

You deserve it.

NOTES:

Exercise *This is where you expand to light weights and moderate activity such as playing a sport, a wilderness hike, or similar. But avoid putting excessive stress on your body and ultimately your system. Your max is not the perceived max. Your max is not putting strain on your system and not allowing your body to work harder than what is possible without exasperating it.*

Probiotics *Depending on progress and current state, this is when you dial back to a maintenance state of 5 billion to 100 billion probiotics daily. You'll know the balance you need.*

HOMEMADE KOMBUCHA

Ingredients

7 cups purified water
2 to 3 tablespoons green tea
2 unbleached tea bags
½ cup coconut sugar
½ gallon glass jar
1 small organic scoby (kombucha starter culture)
½ cup starter liquid (Note: The starter liquid should be from the previous batch, or from a store-bought organic unflavored brand)
Unbleached coffee filter, or cheesecloth
Rubber band
pH test strips
8 (16-ounce) amber glass bottles or Mason jars with tight lids
Small funnel

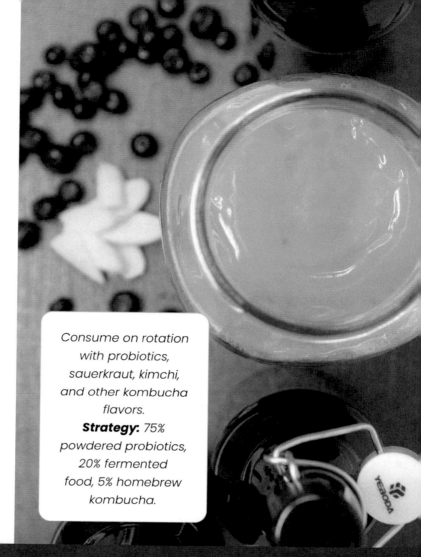

> Consume on rotation with probiotics, sauerkraut, kimchi, and other kombucha flavors.
> **Strategy:** 75% powdered probiotics, 20% fermented food, 5% homebrew kombucha.

Instructions

In a large pot on high heat, bring the water to a boil.
Fill the teabags with the loose tea and secure.
Once the water is boiling, remove the pot from the heat and add the tea bags. Steep for 4 to 5 minutes.
Add the coconut sugar and stir until completely dissolved.
Allow to cool to room temperature, then pour into the glass jar.
Add the starter culture and starter liquid (make sure the tea is cool, to avoid killing the bacteria cultures).
Cover with the coffee filter and secure with the rubber band. Store in a dark, dry, cool place. The ideal temperature should be 70 to 80°.
Leave for 7 to 14 days, until it reaches a pH of 3. Test the brew's pH level with strips.
When ready, remove and carefully place the scoby on a clean plate, being careful to not expose the brew or scoby to foreign bacteria at any time.
Pour ½ cup into a separate ½ gallon jar as the starter liquid for the next batch, then, through a funnel, pour the current batch into glass bottles, leaving 2 inches of head space in each bottle for the fermentation gases.
Add approved ingredients for flavoring (e.g., thinly sliced ginger or turmeric, blueberries, raspberries, or mint), seal, and place back in a dark space for 4 to 5 days.
When the kombucha reaches your desired taste, remove and store in the refrigerator for up to 2 weeks.

If you put you unselfishly first, everything else will healthily live around you.

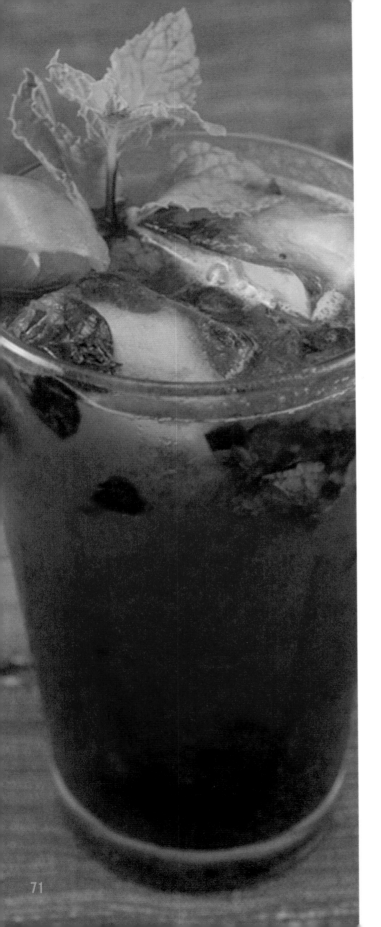

BERRYBUCHA MOCKTAIL

Ingredients

8 to 10 blueberries
Juice of ¼ medium lime
Splash celery juice
3 to 4 fresh mint leaves
6 ounces Homemade Kombucha
(page 70)
3 or 4 purified ice cubes

Garnish

2 fresh mint sprigs
Lime wedge

Instructions

Muddle the blueberries, lime juice, celery juice, and mint leaves in the bottom of a shaker.
Shake for 1 minute.
Add the kombucha and swirl.
Pour over the ice.
Garnish with the mint and lime wedge.

Guar gum: a proven exasperator of the digestive system and trigger of leaky gut. Common in coconut products, alternative milks, frozen treats, and prepackaged drinks.
Avoid it.

STRAWBUCHA MOCKTAIL

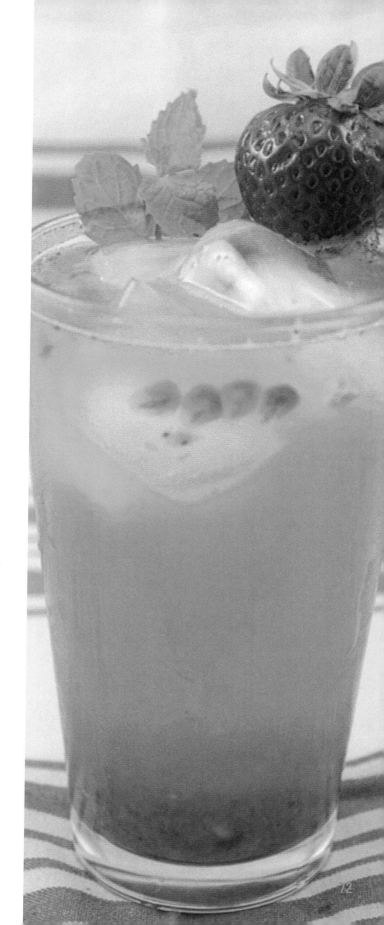

Ingredients

Handful pomegranate seeds

3 or 4 fresh mint leaves

Juice of ½ medium lemon

Splash cranberry juice

½ tablespoon maple syrup

Pinch pink Himalayan sea salt

6 ounces Homemade Kombucha
(page 70)

3 or 4 purified ice cubes

Garnish

2 fresh mint sprigs

1 fresh strawberry

Instructions

Muddle the pomegranate seeds and mint
leaves in the bottom of a shaker.

Combine the lemon juice, cranberry juice,
maple syrup, and salt, and shake for 1 minute.

Add the kombucha and swirl.

Pour over the purified ice.

Garnish with the mint and strawberry.

SPROUTED NUT MILK

Ingredients
1 cup almonds, or walnuts
7 to 8 cups purified water, divided
1 tablespoon apple cider vinegar
3 or 4 dates (omit if avoiding sugar)
Cheesecloth

Optional
1 teaspoon ground cinnamon

Instructions
In a glass container, cover the nuts with 2 cups of purified water (or enough to fully cover them) and the apple cider vinegar. Soak for at least 6 hours and up to overnight to remove any remaining antinutrients. Transfer to a blender or processor and add the remaining purified water and dates. Blend for 3 to 5 minutes or until smooth. If you used almonds or walnuts, strain the mixture into cheesecloth and squeeze the liquids into a glass storage bottle.

Note: Can be stored for up to 1 week.

Nuts, seeds, grains, legumes: Deactivate antinutrients and consume in distant moderation. Only option.

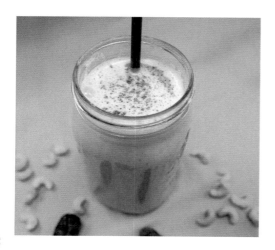

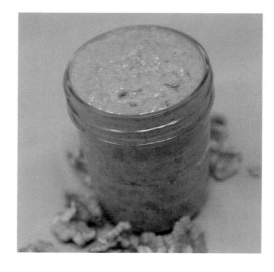

SPROUTED NUT BUTTER

Ingredients
2 cups walnuts or almonds
1 teaspoon coconut oil

Optional
1 teaspoon pink Himalayan sea salt

Instructions
Preheat the oven to 350°.
Spread the nuts evenly on a baking sheet.
Bake for 10 minutes or until lightly golden.
Remove and cool for 10 to 15 minutes.
Transfer to a processor or high-speed blender.
Process for roughly 10 minutes, scraping down the sides occasionally.
When the consistency starts to form a creamy texture, add the oil and salt.
Process for another 5 minutes or until it forms your desired consistency.
Remove and store in an airtight jar in the refrigerator.

Note: Store in the fridge for up to 1 month.

> *The five main "antinutrients" to remember are: phytates, lectins, gluten, tannins, and oxalates.*

CANDIED JEWEL TOAST

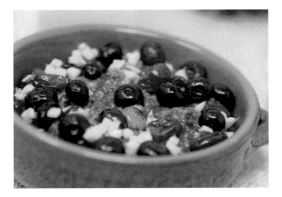

Ingredients
½ tablespoon coconut oil
1 fat jewel sweet potato
1 tablespoon Sprouted Nut Butter
1 medium banana, sliced
½ cup blueberries
Cranberry Sauce (page 23)
Ground cinnamon
Ground ginger

Instructions
In a medium saucepan on medium heat, warm the oil.
Slice the sweet potato into 1-inch-thick rounds from the fattest part.
Cook for 3 to 4 minutes, then flip and cook for another 2 to 3 minutes.
Place on a plate and spread nut butter on each.
Serve topped with the banana, blueberries, and cranberry sauce and sprinkled with cinnamon and ginger.

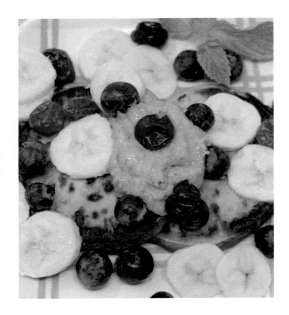

ROYAL OATMEAL

Only glyphosate-free oats!

Ingredients
1/3 cup sprouted oats
2 cups purified water

Toppings
1 teaspoon ground cinnamon
½ teaspoon ground turmeric
½ cup fresh blueberries or 1 medium banana
Spoonful Cranberry Sauce (page 23)
1 scoop (20 g) collagen peptides
½ tablespoon carob powder
1 teaspoon manuka honey
1 tablespoon minced peeled fresh ginger

Optional
Handful of nuts or ¼ cup nut milk,
plus more nut milk for serving

Instructions
In a medium pot on medium heat, combine the oats and 2 cups of purified water.
Bring the mixture to a simmer and cook for 15 to 20 minutes, until the water fully absorbs.
Scoop into a bowl and top with your desired toppings.
Drizzle with nut milk (if using) to reach your desired consistency.

Antioxidants? Compounds that help protect cells from oxidants. (Anti the oxidants) Oxidants? Oxygen turns to oxidation, which turns to free radicals, which develops into disease.

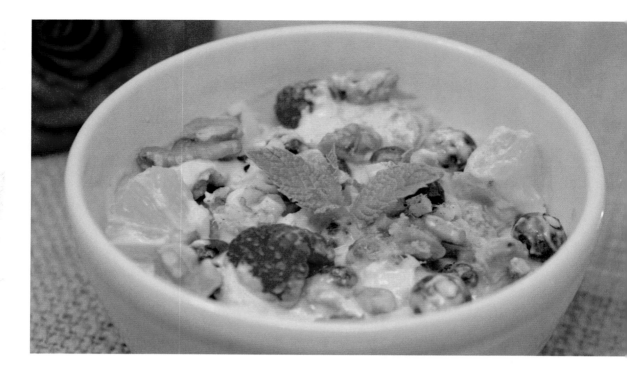

MARILYN'S FRUIT SALAD

Keep focused on your goals and good things will happen.

Ingredients

3 fresh mint leaves

Blueberries

Raspberries

½ medium orange, sliced

1 teaspoon ground cinnamon

1 tablespoon minced peeled fresh ginger

½ cup Better Belly Yogurt (page 78)

Optional

½ cup soaked walnuts

2 teaspoons apple cider vinegar

1 cup purified water

Instructions

If using walnuts, soak them in the apple cider vinegar and purified water in a glass container for at least 6 hours and up to overnight.

Strain, rinse, and dry the walnuts.

Finely chop the mint.

Combine all the ingredients together in a bowl and gently mix.

When new conditions arise, adjust. You can't be naïve to change. Your body is changing every moment and healing lies in your ability to stay present with the changes. Common underlying scenarios: avoiding starchy carbohydrates, fructose dominate foods, Candida triggers, and FODMAP foods (pages 8-12).

COCONANERS PANCAKES

Ingredients

Olive, coconut, or avocado oil

1 medium banana

1 cup Sprouted Nut Milk (page 73)

1 teaspoon lemon juice

½ cup coconut flour

1 teaspoon ground cinnamon

1 scoop (20 g) collagen peptides

½ tablespoon carob powder

Topping

Fresh strawberries or other
approved fruit

Maple syrup

Instructions

Heat a griddle or pan on medium heat and coat with oil.

In a bowl, mash the banana. Add the nut milk and lemon juice and stir until thoroughly mixed.

Add the flour, cinnamon, collagen peptides, and carob powder and mix until a pancake consistency forms.

Pour 2- to 3-inch pancakes onto the griddle and cook until lightly golden brown. Flip and finish cooking.

WHIPPED CREAM

Ingredients

1 cup walnuts or almonds

1¼ cups purified water, divided

2 teaspoons apple cider vinegar

1 tablespoon manuka honey or maple syrup

1 teaspoon vanilla extract

1/8 teaspoon pink Himalayan sea salt

Instructions

Soak the nuts in 1 cup of purified water and the apple cider vinegar for at least 6 hours and up to 24 hours.

Strain, wash, and dry the nuts.

In a blender or food processor, combine the nuts, honey, vanilla, and salt.

Process on a slow to medium setting, slowly adding the remaining water until a smooth cream consistency forms (scrape the sides a time or two in the process).

Transfer to a bowl and chill for 1 to 2 hours.

Did you stretch today? Do it!

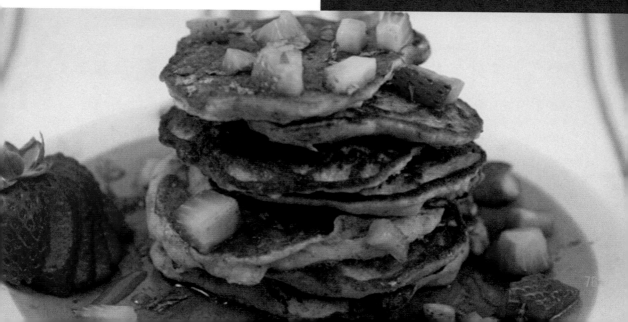

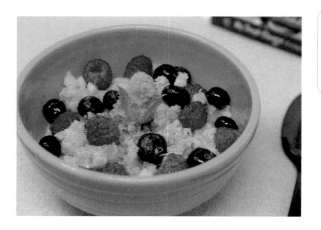

CAULIFLOWER RICE PUDDING

Ingredients

1 medium to large cauliflower, cut into florets
1 cup nut milk, plus more for topping
1 cup purified water
2 teaspoons ground cinnamon
1 tablespoon minced peeled fresh ginger

Topping

½ cup approved fruit
1 tablespoon manuka honey or
1 tablespoon maple syrup

Instructions

In a processor, process the cauliflower for a few seconds, until a little bigger than rice.
Transfer to a medium pot on medium-high heat.
Add the nut milk, water, cinnamon, and ginger.
Bring to a boil, then reduce the heat to low.
Simmer for 10 to 12 minutes, stirring occasionally, until the rice is tender and the mixture has reached a pudding texture.
Add your desired toppings and serve warm or chill in the fridge.

PROBIOTIC PUDDING

Ingredients

1 medium sweet potato (or squash)
½ cup Sprouted Nut Milk (page 73)
½ to 1 tablespoon honey or maple syrup
1 scoop (20 g) collagen peptides
Ground cinnamon
1/2 tablespoon ground ginger
1 (10-billion) serving probiotics
1 piece or ½ cup approved fruit

Optional

Want to make it "cocoa" pudding? Add...
½ to 1 tablespoon carob powder

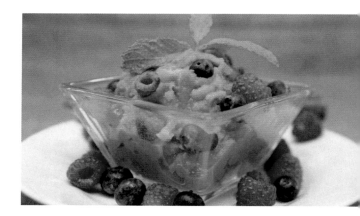

Instructions

Preheat the oven to 375°.
Bake the sweet potato for 45 minutes or until soft.
Remove the skin and refrigerate until cold.
In a blender, blend together the sweet potato and nut milk.
Blending on the lowest setting, add the honey, collagen peptides, cinnamon, ground ginger, and carob powder (if using).
Transfer to a bowl and gently mix in the probiotics.
Top with the fruit and gently stir it in.

BETTER BELLY YOGURT

Ingredients

[ ] cup cashews
[ ]urified water for soaking, plus ¾ cup
[ ] teaspoon pink Himalayan sea salt
[ ] tablespoon apple cider vinegar
[ ] (10-billion) serving of probiotics
[ ] tablespoon psyllium husk powder

Toppings

[ ] piece or ½ cup approved fruit of choice
[ ]prouted nuts, coconut chips, carob powder,
[ ]ound cinnamon, ground or minced ginger,
[ ]ound turmeric, manuka honey, maple syrup,
[ ]d anything else in this book that your happy
[ ]art desires.

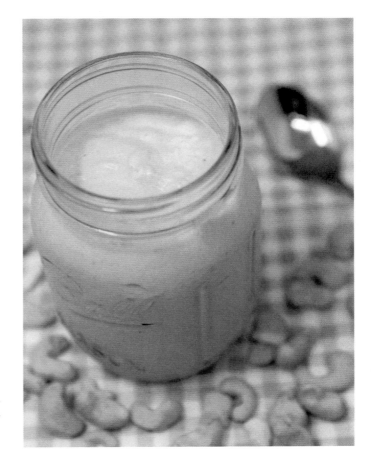

Instructions

[ ]oak the cashews in purified water with the salt and apple cider vinegar for
[ ] least 6 hours and up to overnight.
[ ]reheat the oven to 100°. If that's not possible, preheat it to its lowest temp
[ ]d turn the oven off when it reaches 100°. Do not open the oven door.
[ ]rain and rinse the cashews and transfer to a processor or blender.
[ ]dd ¾ cup of purified water and blend until smooth.
[ ]dd the probiotics and psyllium husk powder and stir until smooth.
[ ]ansfer the mixture to a sterilized quart-size mason jar. (Note: You can
[ ]erilize your jar by boiling it in water. Make sure to let it cool to room
[ ]mperature before adding the yogurt.)
[ ]ace the jar, without its lid, in the oven. Turn on the oven light.
[ ]eave the jar in the oven for 12 to 24 hours (the longer, the tarter). Very
[ ]nportant: Do not open the oven during this time. It's vital to keep all heat
[ ]ntained. The sealed oven with the light will stay at about 105°, perfect to
[ ]rment the mix.
[ ]emove the yogurt from the oven and stir well.
[ ]over and let it chill in the fridge until completely chilled, 3 to 5 hours.
[ ]ote: If after chilling, the texture isn't smooth, toss it in the processor until
[ ] reaches your desired creaminess, and store in the fridge for up to 2 weeks.

Your breath is your anchor.

Cashews increase the risk for mold exposure significantly. Treat them and consume them with caution and awareness.

SPECIAL OCCASIONS COOKIES

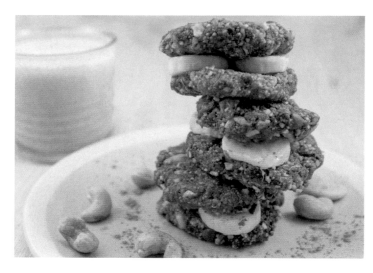

Ingredients

1 cup sprouted walnuts
¼ cup almonds or cashews
1 medium banana
Purified water
1 tablespoon apple cider vinegar
4 pitted dates
1 tablespoon coconut oil
1 tablespoon ground cinnamon
1 tablespoon carob powder

Instructions

Soak the walnuts and almonds (or cashews) in purified water and the apple cider vinegar for at least 6 hours and up to overnight. Strain and wash the nuts.
Combine them with the dates in a processor and process until small pieces of dough start to form.
Add the coconut oil, cinnamon, and carob powder.
Mix on medium until a dough completely forms.
Refrigerate for 20 to 30 minutes.
Form into cookies.

BUTTER BALLS

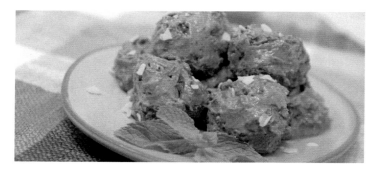

Ingredients

1 cup sprouted walnuts
¼ cup almonds or cashews
1 medium banana
Purified water
1 tablespoon apple cider vinegar
4 pitted dates
1 tablespoon coconut oil
1 tablespoon ground cinnamon
1 tablespoon carob powder

Instructions

In a medium bowl, mash the banana.
Add the collagen peptides, coconut oil, maple syrup, turmeric, and cinnamon and mix thoroughly.
Add the nut butter and thoroughly mix.
Fold in the coconut flakes, blueberries, ginger, and cranberry sauce.
Cover the bowl and place in the freezer for 30 minutes.
Mold to your desired size.
Store in the freezer for at least 1 hour.

ANTS ON A LOG

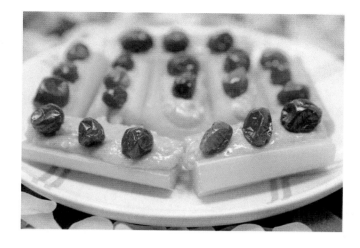

Ingredients

Celery, washed, dried, and cut into
3- to 5-inch lengths
Sprouted Nut Butter (page 74)
Cranberries
¼ cup purified water

Instructions

Fill the celery trench with nut butter.
In a small pot on medium heat, combine the cranberries and
water, and lightly simmer until the cranberries soften and the
water evaporates.
Allow to cool, and add the ants to the logs.

No more missing days and life's best moments because of that "something" you did something about! Be proud of that.

TEETH MARK'S CHEESE

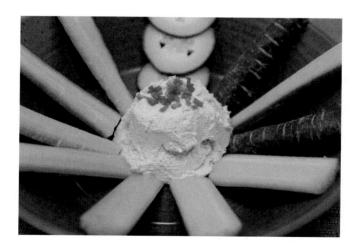

Ingredients

1 cup walnuts or almonds
Purified water
1 tablespoon apple cider vinegar
½ tablespoon lemon juice
½ teaspoon pink Himalayan salt
¼ cup water

Instructions

Soak the nuts in purified water and the apple cider vinegar for at least 4 hours and up to overnight.
Strain and rinse the nuts.
Combine the nuts, lemon juice, and salt in a food processor.
Pulse until evenly combined.
Slowly add the water until smooth or it reaches your desired creaminess.

This isn't about quitting cold turkey. It's about minimizing the waves of the moments that cause regression until they are worked out of the days. By addressing, understanding, adjusting, incorporating, and gradually moving away from the problematic situation.

SQUASH SOUP

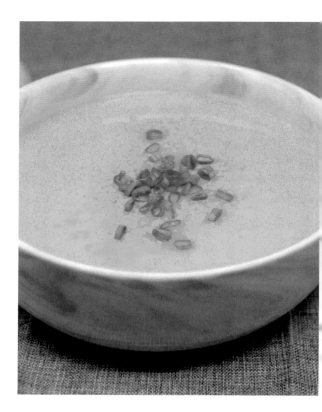

Ingredients

1 medium to large baked butternut squash
(page 14)

1 tablespoons olive oil

4 cups Bone Broth (page 19)

1 tablespoon manuka honey (or maple syrup)

2 teaspoons ground turmeric

1 teaspoon pink Himalayan sea salt

½ avocado

¼ cup chopped scallion

Optional

½ cup diced sweet onion

2 garlic cloves, minced

Instructions

In a large pot on medium heat, warm the olive oil.

If using the onions and garlic, add them to the pot and cook until soft, 3 to 5 minutes.

Add the squash flesh, broth, honey, turmeric, and salt.

Stir to combine.

Reduce the heat to low and let the soup simmer, covered, for 25 to 30 minutes.

Remove the soup from the heat, remove the lid, and let cool for 20 minutes.

Working in batches, puree the soup in a processer or blender until it reaches your desired creaminess.

Serve topped with the avocado and scallion.

HONEY-CIDER DRESSING

"It's just a little bit" is still something. It's still regression. After how hard you've been working?

Ingredients

1/3 cup olive oil

1 tablespoon apple cider vinegar

1 tablespoon lemon juice

1 tablespoon coconut aminos

2 teaspoons manuka honey or maple syrup

½ teaspoon grated fresh peeled ginger

½ teaspoon pink Himalayan sea salt

Optional

1 garlic clove, minced

Instructions

Combine all the ingredients in a glass jar
and shake until evenly combined

HEAVENLY SUSHI ROLL

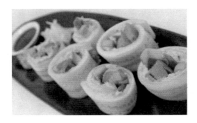

Ingredients

1 large cucumber, peeled and sliced into long strips
1/3 cup Citrus Artichoke Hummus (page 53)
1 medium carrot, cut into 1-inch matchsticks
½ avocado, sliced
Wild-caught salmon
½ tablespoon chopped fresh dill
3 or 4 lemon wedges

Sides

Coconut aminos
Fresh wasabi
Fresh pickled ginger

Optional

Salmon or tuna, heavy metal tested and in small portions in respect to your weekly intake.

Instructions

Dry the cucumber with paper towels.
On a flat surface, spread the hummus on each cucumber strip.
Evenly lay the carrot, avocado, and salmon over the hummus.
Tightly roll each cucumber strip (if you're having trouble keeping them rolled, a toothpick works wonders).
Stick a small sprig of dill into the center of each roll.
Squeeze lemon juice on top.
Note: Keep the cucumber and hummus base, then mix and match any desirable ingredient from the foods lists. Keep it fresh by getting creative!

MAHALO BOATS

Ingredients

6 ounces salmon, or cubed roasted butternut squash (page 14)
½ cup Avocado Mayo (page 25)
1 teaspoon ground turmeric
2 teaspoons coconut aminos
½ tablespoon minced peeled fresh ginger
1 tablespoon lime juice
1 head romaine heart or endive
¼ cup fresh pineapple chunks
1 scallion, thinly sliced
1/4 cup sliced carrots
¼ cup thinly sliced cucumber

Dressing

Honey-Cider Dressing

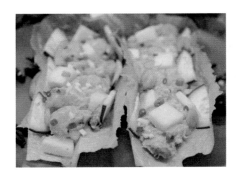

Instructions

Strain the salmon and combine in a bowl with the mayo, turmeric, coconut aminos, ginger, and lime juice.
Stir until evenly mixed.
Wash and plate the romaine leaves.
Scoop your desired salmon mixture onto the leaves.
Top with the pineapple, scallion, carrots, and cucumber.
Drizzle with dressing.

Inflammation in the gut increases with age as intestinal reliability gradually declines. The more chronic the inflammation, the faster the aging process. Ultimately causing the gut to become permeable and leaky over time, depending on exposure. The result: cancerous diseases.

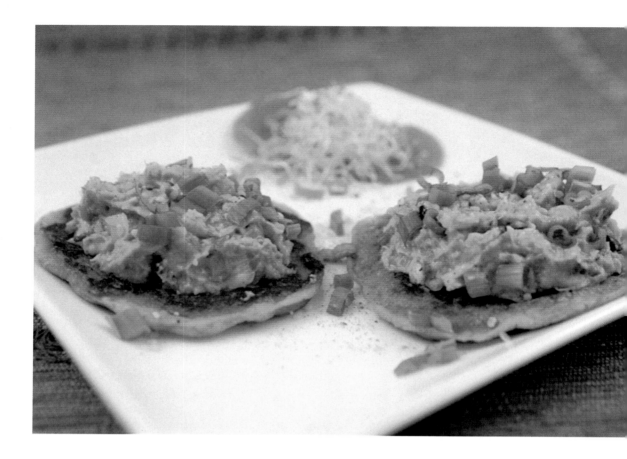

OMEGA DIP

Ingredients

1 teaspoon olive oil
¼ cup thinly sliced leeks (green part only)
¼ cup diced carrots
¼ cup diced celery
2 medium avocados
1 tablespoon Deactivated Beans (page 56)
½ tablespoon coconut aminos
½ tablespoon minced fresh dill
2 tablespoons chopped unpitted black olives
¼ cup sauerkraut
1 (6- to 8-ounce) serving cooked salmon
¼ cup microgreens
1 teaspoon ground turmeric
Pinch pink Himalayan sea salt
Juice of 1 lime
Zest of ½ lime

Topping

2 tablespoons thinly sliced scallions
Broccoli sprouts
3 to 5 watercress leaves, chopped

Optional

If flatbread is too heavy for your system, replace with Crepe Roll-ups (page 50), or enjoy as a dip with Savory Plantain Chips (page 33) or in a collard green wrap.

Instructions

In a medium pan on medium heat, warm the olive oil.
Add the leeks, carrots, and celery and sauté for 3 to 5 minutes, until light golden brown.
Mash the avocados in a bowl.
Add the sauté mixture, beans, coconut aminos, dill, olives, sauerkraut, salmon, microgreens, turmeric, salt, lime juice, and lime zest.
Gently mix until thoroughly combined.
Cover and place in the fridge for 15 to 20 minutes.
Serve topped with the scallions, sprouts, and watercress.

FLATBREAD

Ingredients

Avocado oil cooking spray
½ cup sprouted corn flour or coconut flour
2 tablespoons psyllium husk powder
2 teaspoons rosemary needles
¼ teaspoon pink Himalayan sea salt
¼ cup melted coconut oil
1 cup purified water, boiling
1 tablespoon olive oil
Pesto

Instructions

Preheat the oven to 400°. Line a baking sheet with foil and spray with oil.

In a medium bowl, combine the corn flour, psyllium husk powder, rosemary, and salt and stir together until well combined.

Slowly pour in the melted coconut oil and hot water, stirring until a dough forms.

Allow to cool until the dough can be handled.

Split into 4 or 5 balls.

Before the dough cools completely, roll the balls into flatbread between two sheets of parchment paper.

Baste with the olive oil and place on the baking sheet.

Bake for 8 to 12 minutes, until crispy brown and the edges are very crispy.

Spread the flatbread with pesto.

PESTO

Ingredients

1½ cups pressed basil or arugula
¼ cup walnuts
1 teaspoon apple cider vinegar
1 cup purified water
⅓ cup olive oil
4 garlic cloves
¼ teaspoon pink Himalayan sea salt
1 tablespoon lemon juice

Instructions

Combine all the ingredients in a processor and blend until it reaches your preferred consistency.

Stop livin' by the negative statistics. Start believin' in your success.

Mix omegas with a blend of healthy digestible fiber to reduce inflammation in key parts of the body, like the large intestine.

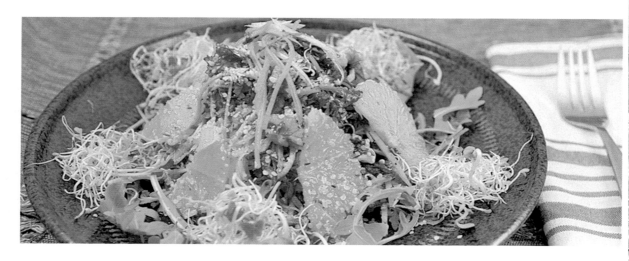

CITRUS SALAD W/ MAPLE LEMON VINAIGRETTE

Ingredients

¼ cup walnuts

½ cup purified water (enough to cover nuts)

1 teaspoon apple cider vinegar

1 Roasted Beet (page 14), diced

1 cup arugula

¼ cup shaven multicolored carrots

⅓ avocado

½ grapefruit, or 1 orange, cut into segments

Topping

¼ cup broccoli sprouts

Maple Lemon Vinaigrette

Instructions

In a glass storage container, combine the walnuts, water, and apple cider vinegar. Soak for at least 6 hours and up to overnight. Drain, wash, and dry the walnuts.

Preheat the oven to 425°.

Make a bed of arugula on a plate.

Cover with the beets, carrots, and avocado, crushing the walnuts as you sprinkle them on.

Top with the grapefruit and sprouts and drizzle with dressing.

Optional

This salad also goes well topped with baked butternut squash w/veggies (page 14).

MAPLE LEMON VINAIGRETTE

Ingredients

2 tablespoons olive oil

1 tablespoon lemon juice

1 teaspoon maple syrup

Pinch pink Himalayan sea salt

Instructions

Whisk together the dressing ingredients in a bowl.

Store in a glass jar.

SPRING SALAD W/RASPBERRY WALNUT VINAIGRETTE

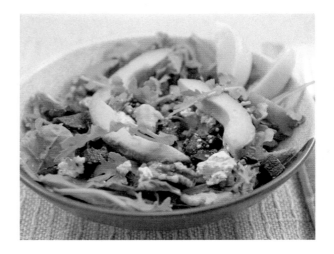

Ingredients

1 cup arugula

1 teaspoon lemon juice

1 medium roasted beet (page 14), diced

1/3 avocado, sliced

1 tablespoon Teeth Mark's Cheese (page 80)

1 tablespoon hemp seeds

Raspberry Walnut Vinaigrette

Optional

Handful walnuts

Purified water

1 tablespoon apple cider vinegar

Instructions

If using walnuts, soak them in a glass container with purified water and the apple cider vinegar for at least 6 hours and up to overnight. Strain, wash, and dry the walnuts (if using).

In a small bowl, top the arugula with the lemon juice. Refrigerate for 20 to 30 minutes to allow it to "cook."

Remove the salad from the refrigerator, and top with the beet, avocado, Teeth Mark's Cheese, walnuts (if using), and hemp seeds.

Drizzle with vinaigrette.

RASPBERRY WALNUT VINAIGRETTE

Ingredients

½ cup olive oil

½ tablespoons apple cider vinegar

½ cup raspberries, thawed if frozen

1 tablespoon lemon juice

½ teaspoon pink Himalayan sea salt

1½ teaspoons manuka honey, or maple syrup

Optional

2 tablespoons walnuts

Purified water

1 tablespoon apple cider vinegar

Instructions

If using walnuts, soak them in a glass container with purified water and the apple cider vinegar for at least 6 hours and up to overnight.

Mash the raspberries in a small bowl.

Strain, wash, dry, and crumble the walnuts (if using).

Combine all the ingredients in a glass jar and shake until evenly mixed.

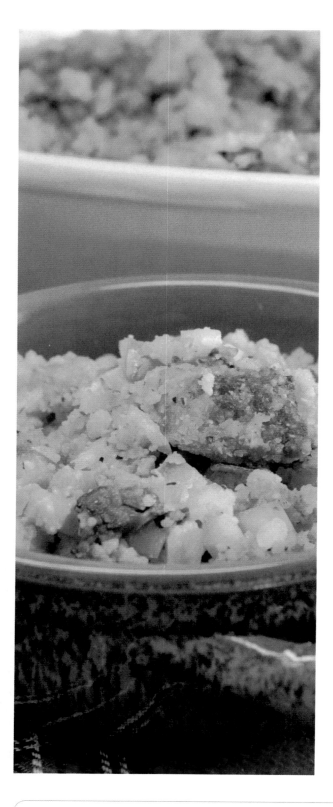

HOLIDAY STUFFING

Ingredients

1 cup cranberries
1 tablespoon purified water
½ cup diced celery
½ cup diced leeks
½ cup diced mushrooms
1 teaspoon minced fresh thyme
½ tablespoon minced fresh sage
½ tablespoon minced peeled fresh ginger
1 tablespoon ground turmeric
1 cup Bone Broth (page 19)
2 tablespoons olive oil
2 pinches pink Himalayan sea salt
Flatbread (page 84), broken into small pieces

Instructions

Preheat the oven to 350°.
In a small pan on medium heat, combine
the cranberries and water.
Cook until the water has been fully
absorbed or evaporated.
Transfer to a glass baking dish and add
the celery, leeks, mushrooms, thyme,
sage, ginger, turmeric, broth, oil, and salt.
Mix well.
If dry, slowly add more bone broth until
it reaches your desired creaminess.
Spread the mixture evenly.
Top with the flatbread (imagine a
"crumble" topping).
Bake for 20 to 30 minutes, until the top is
golden brown.

The only thing you should ever regret is the time you spend regretting. Cherish every holiday, every meal, and every person in-between.

PUMPKIN PIE

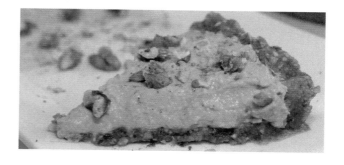

Ingredients

Crust

1 cup plus 2 tablespoons coconut flour

½ cup olive oil

2 to 3 tablespoons purified water

Optional

½ cup ground sprouted walnuts, processed into small pieces

3 or 4 pitted dates, processed into small pieces

Filling

1¾ cups (1 can) pumpkin puree

½ cup coconut milk

1 tablespoon lemon juice

3 tablespoons maple syrup

1 teaspoon ground cinnamon

1 teaspoon ground ginger

Pinch pink Himalayan sea salt

Instructions

Crust

Preheat the oven to 375°.

Combine the coconut flour, oil, and water in a bowl and hand mix until it forms a dough-like consistency, adding the water slowly as you go.

Add the walnuts and dates (if using) and stir until evenly mixed. (Remember, nuts are a once in a while treat).

In a 6-inch pie plate, press the dough to form an even crust. (If using 8-or 9-inch pie dish, double or triple the ingredients respectively. But be aware of overconsumption!!)

Filling

In a food processor, combine all the ingredients.

Blend until combined (avoid overblending into a puree).

Spoon the filling into the crust and smooth until even.

Place in the oven for 20 to 30 minutes and let cool.

TURMERIC LATTE

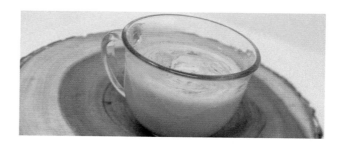

Ingredients

½ inch fresh peeled turmeric or 1 teaspoon ground turmeric

¼ inch fresh ginger, peeled

1 teaspoon manuka honey

1 cup Sprouted Nut Milk (page 73)

½ cup purified water

Pinch pink Himalayan sea salt

½ teaspoon ground cinnamon

Instructions

Combine the turmeric, ginger, honey, nut milk, water, and salt in a processor or blender and blend until smooth or frothy texture.

Pour the liquid into a small pot on medium heat and warm to your desired temperature.

Pour into a mug and garnish with the cinnamon.

THE SIGNATURE

Ingredients

¾ ounce fresh lime juice
1 ounce Ginger Simple Syrup (page 36)
1 fresh mint sprig
Purified ice cubes
4½ ounces Homemade Kombucha (page 70)
Copper mug

Garnish

Lime wedge
2 or 3 fresh mint leaves
Candied Ginger (page 36)

Instructions

In a shaker, combine the lime juice and
simple syrup and shake for 10 seconds.
Add the mint to the shaker and muddle.
Add 2 purified ice cubes.
Shake for 1 minute.
Add the kombucha and gently swirl.
Strain into a copper mug (rocks glass if
you must) filled with purified ice cubes.
Garnish with the lime wedge, mint leaves,
and a piece of candied ginger.

Peer pressure persuasion.
That was the old you.
This is your Signature.

*When it comes to alcohol, there
isn't a perfect solution other than
elimination. Every other choice that
includes alcohol causes inflammation
and exposes regression.*

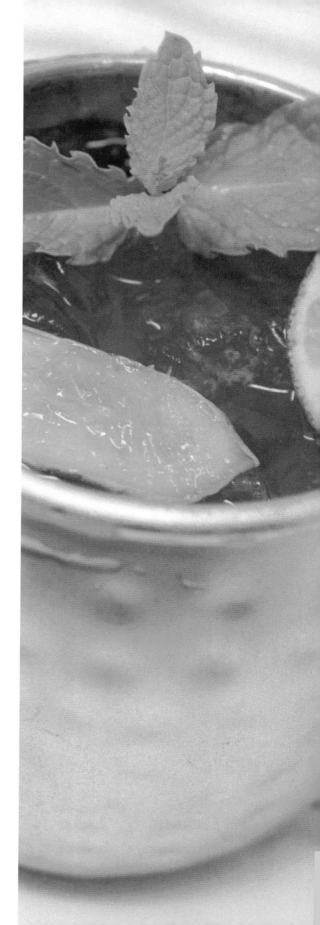

DESSERT...

The sweet treat of success is the only dessert you'll ever need and the only one you'll find in this book. After all the hard work of each day that brought the deliciousness of this moment, you're going to ruin it by eating a bowl of sugar and detrimental ingredients just before bed? That logic puts every day on repeat.

Instead, pour some warm water, kick your feet up, have a conversation of substance or some music of unwinding spirit, and smile.

For one more day forward.
For another step in the right direction.
For you.
For relief.
For proving yourself right.
And for more days here, with the ones who mean the most.

You've achieved what was once said to be impossible.
Congratulations.

No matter what comes next, remember what got you here.

And, always,
stay willing.

Recipes help.
Everything together, heals.

INDEX

INDEX

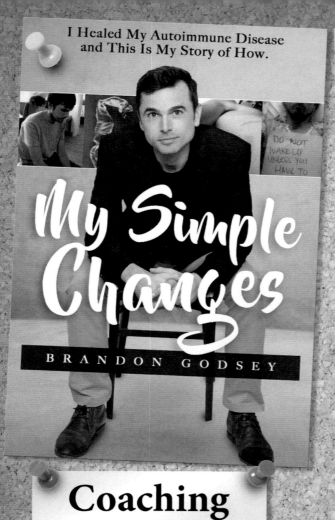

I Healed My Autoimmune Disease and This Is My Story of How.

My Simple Changes Book

My Simple Changes

BRANDON GODSEY

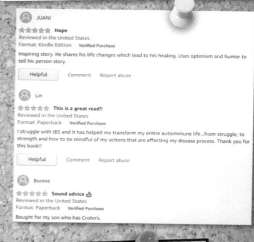

JUANI
★★★★★ Hope
Reviewed in the United States
Format: Kindle Edition   Verified Purchase
Inspiring story. He shares his life changes which lead to his healing. Uses optimism and humor to tell his person story.

Helpful   Comment   Report abuse

Lin
★★★★★ This is a great read!!
Reviewed in the United States
Format: Paperback   Verified Purchase
I struggle with IBS and it has helped me transform my entire autoimmune life...from struggle, to strength and how to be mindful of my actions that are affecting my disease process. Thank you for this book!!

Helpful   Comment   Report abuse

Bonnie
★★★★★ Sound advice 👍
Reviewed in the United States
Format: Paperback   Verified Purchase
Bought for my son who has Crohn's.

Coaching

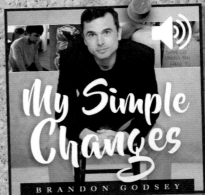

My Simple Changes

BRANDON GODSEY

Author Narrated Audiobook

- Identifying underlying conditions
- Reducing your toxic load
- Building meal plans
- Your product replacements
- To Schedule, Contact:
  Brandon@MySimpleChanges.com

Ready for the next phase of the Changes?
www.MySimpleChanges.com

     My Simple Changes

Made in the USA
Middletown, DE
28 December 2020